Architecture of the Human Journey

The Energetic Body
(Book 3)

Traditional Chinese Medicine, Qi Theory, and Energetic Anatomy

By Jim Moltzan

Disclaimer

This book is intended for informational and educational purposes only. It is not a substitute for professional medical, psychological, or mental health treatment. Nothing in this book should be interpreted as medical advice, mental health diagnosis, clinical intervention, or a guarantee of outcome. Readers experiencing significant emotional distress, trauma symptoms, or health concerns should consult a qualified healthcare or mental health professional.

The practices and concepts presented herein are offered as general guidance. The author does not promise or imply any specific results, nor is the author responsible for any adverse outcomes arising from the use or misuse of the information contained in this book. Use the material at your own discretion and risk.

The author has made every effort to ensure accuracy and completeness. However, the author makes no representations or warranties regarding the applicability, fitness, or completeness of the content for any individual reader.

ISBN: 978-1-958837-57-3

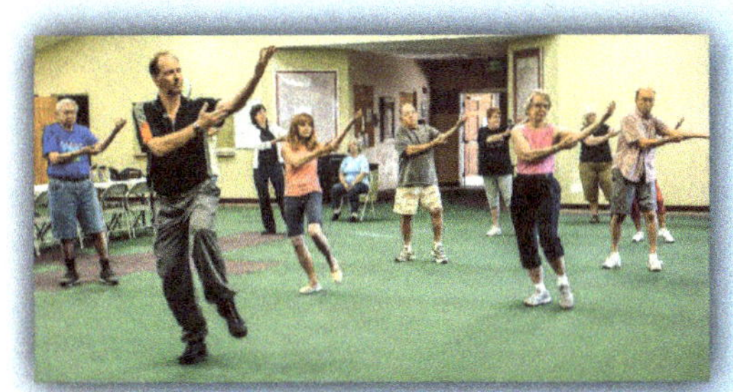
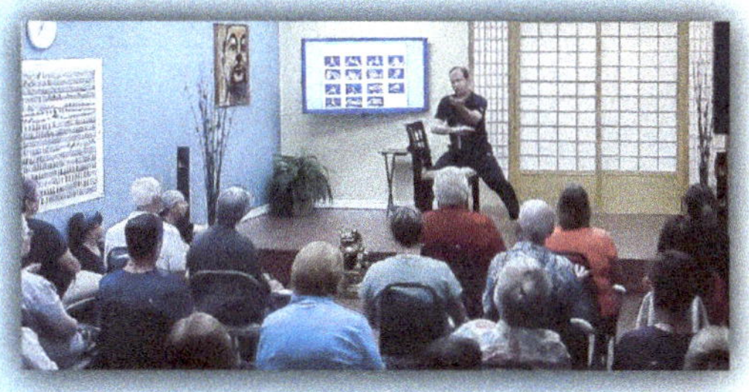
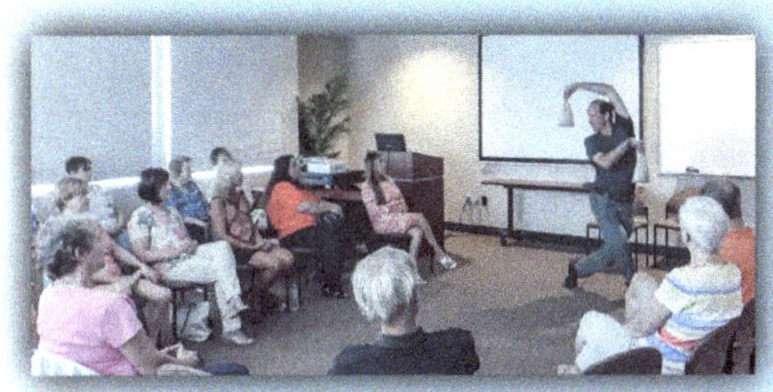
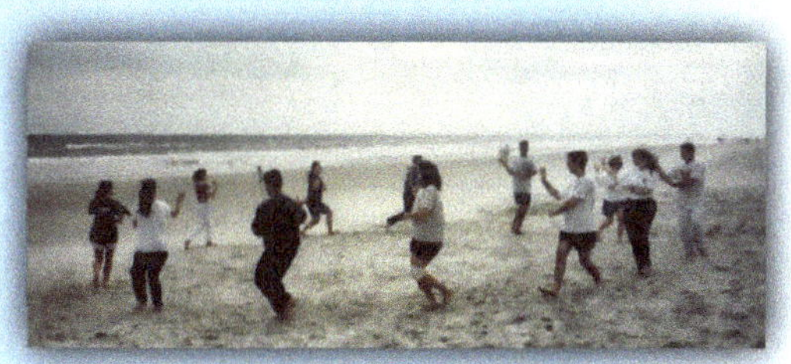
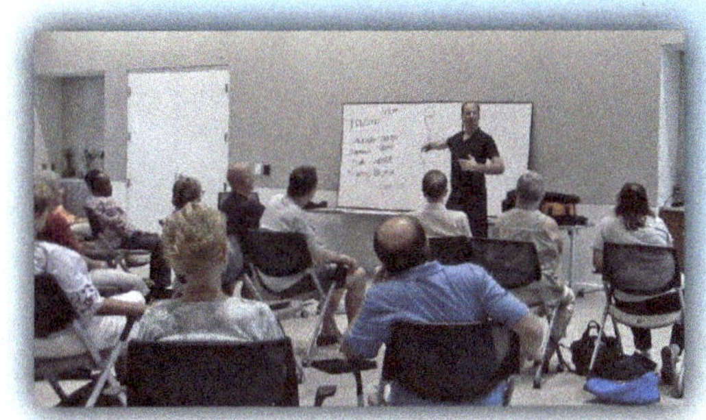
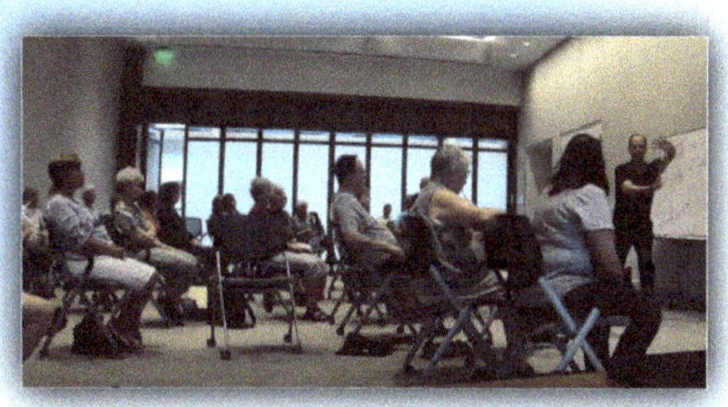
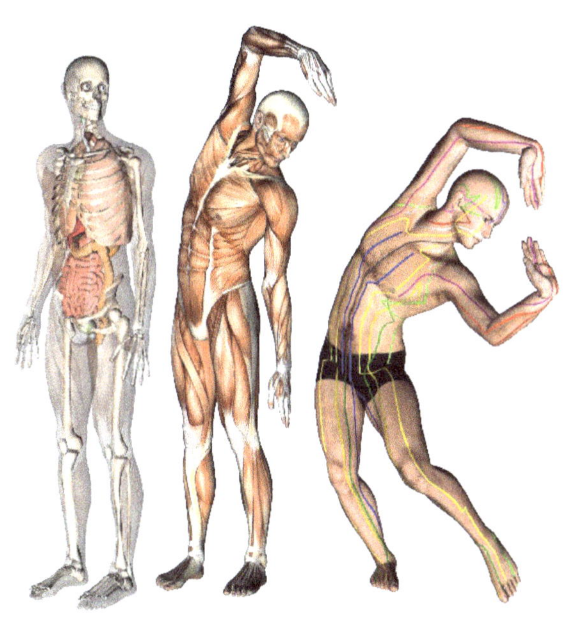

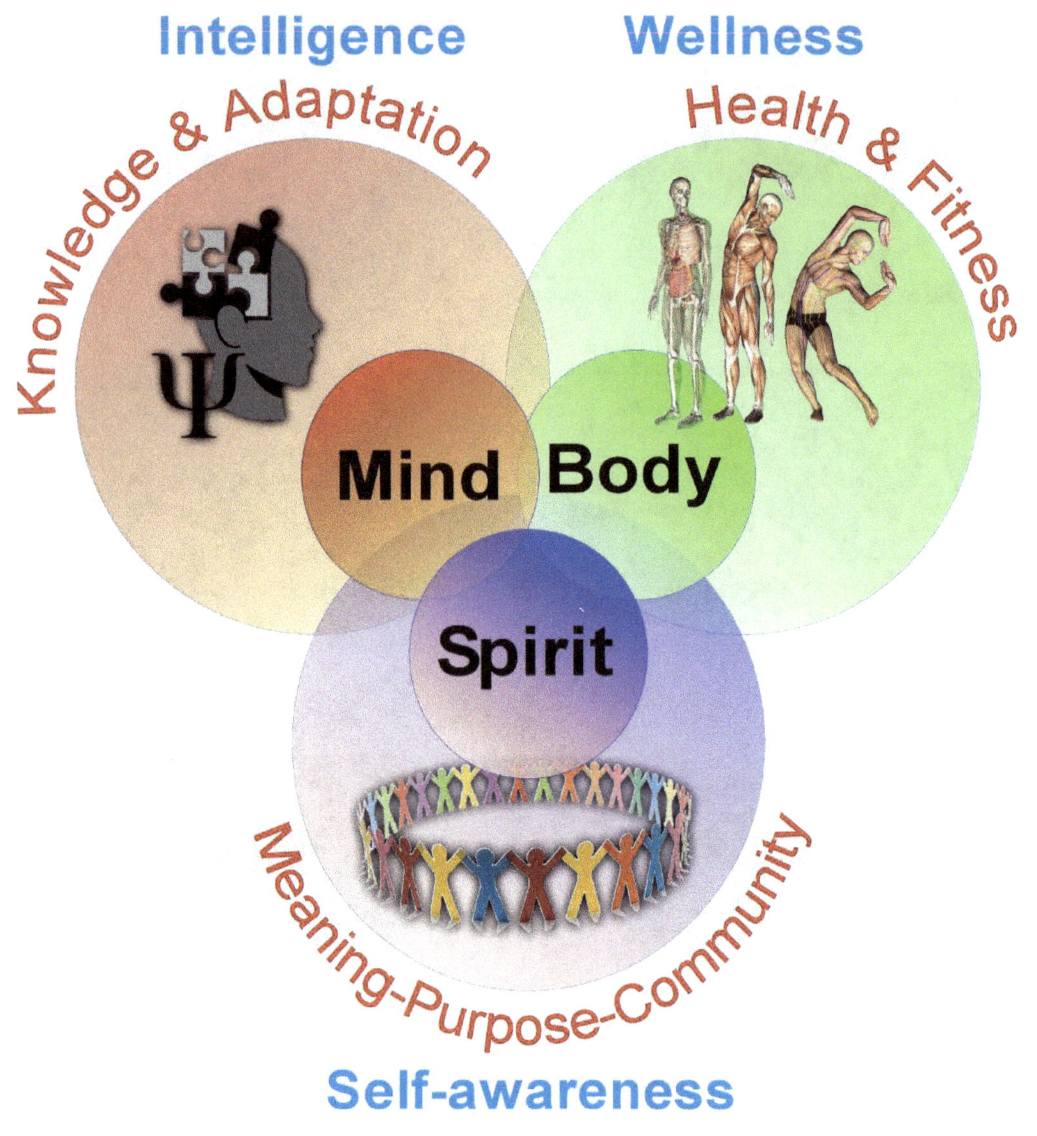

We become the architects of our lives once safety, awareness, and agency are restored.

Table of Contents

Preface: Understanding the Energetic Body

The concept of an "energetic body" has been present across cultures for thousands of years. Whether described as Qi in Traditional Chinese Medicine, Prana in Ayurveda, or vital force in other traditions, the underlying idea is consistent: human life is sustained not only by physical structures, but by dynamic processes that regulate, animate, and integrate those structures into a living system.

In modern Western science, this language has evolved into terms such as nervous system regulation, circulation, and biochemical signaling. While the terminology differs, the essential observation remains unchanged. The human organism functions as an interconnected, adaptive network, constantly responding to both internal and external conditions.

This book explores that integration through the lens of Traditional Chinese Medicine (TCM), while also drawing connections to contemporary understanding in physiology, movement science, and human behavior. The intention is not to position one system as superior to another, but to demonstrate how these perspectives can complement one another when viewed through a broader, integrative framework.

At its core, the energetic model is a way of describing relationships: between breath and nervous system regulation, movement and circulation, emotion and physiological response, and awareness and behavior. These relationships are not abstract concepts. They are observable, trainable, and measurable through direct experience.

Throughout this book, you will encounter foundational ideas such as *Qi*, the meridian system, and the Three Treasures of *Jing, Qi,* and *Shen*. These concepts are presented not as rigid doctrines, but as functional models that help organize perception and guide practice. They offer a way of understanding how balance is maintained, how disruption occurs, and how restoration can be cultivated over time.

You will also be introduced to practical methods drawn from Qigong, breathwork, joint mobility, and traditional therapeutic approaches. These practices are not isolated techniques, but interconnected tools designed to restore rhythm, improve circulation, and support internal coherence.

A central theme throughout this work is that health is not merely the absence of illness, but the presence of adaptability, or the ability to respond to stress, recover efficiently, and maintain stability within constant change.

From this perspective, the energetic body is not something separate or mystical. It is a way of understanding how the body functions as a whole, an integrated system shaped by breath, movement, awareness, and time.

Acknowledgments: Lineage, Experience, and Shared Practice

This book reflects not only years of personal study, practice, and teaching, but also the influence of many individuals, traditions, and lived experiences that have shaped my understanding of the energetic body. While the material is presented through my own lens, it is rooted in a much larger continuum of knowledge that spans generations.

I am grateful to the teachers who introduced me to the principles of movement, breath, and internal cultivation. Some offered direct instruction, while others taught through observation, correction, or example. In many cases, the most valuable lessons came not only from what was explained clearly, but from what required time, effort, and experience to understand. Each of these influences contributed to the gradual refinement of both my practice and perspective.

To my students, past and present, I offer sincere appreciation. Your questions, challenges, and commitment to learning have continually shaped how I teach and how I continue to grow. The process of guiding others often reveals the practical strengths and limitations of any method, and your willingness to engage in that process has helped ground this work in real-world application rather than theory alone.

I also acknowledge the enduring traditions from which many of these concepts originate, particularly those within Traditional Chinese Medicine, Taoist philosophy, and the internal martial arts. These systems have persisted because they are based on careful observation of natural patterns and human experience. While interpretations may evolve over time, their foundational insights remain both relevant and adaptable.

To colleagues and peers working in the fields of health, movement, and human development, your continued efforts to explore, question, and integrate knowledge across disciplines contribute to a broader and more meaningful understanding of the human condition. The intersection of traditional wisdom and modern science offers a valuable opportunity for clarity rather than conflict.

Finally, I recognize the quieter aspects of this process in the hours of practice, reflection, revision, and persistence that are not visible on the page but are essential to its creation. This work is as much a product of that internal process as it is of external influence.

If this book provides clarity, direction, or practical value, it stands as a shared effort shaped by many contributions along the way.

Author's Note: An Embodied Perspective on Energy and Practice

My understanding of the energetic body has developed over more than four decades of study, practice, and teaching within the fields of martial arts, breath training, and holistic health. What began as a physical pursuit gradually evolved into a deeper exploration of how the body, mind, and internal processes are inseparably connected.

Early in my training, much of the focus was placed on external form in posture, strength, conditioning, and repetition. Over time, it became clear that these elements, while important, represent only one layer of development. As attention shifted toward breath, internal awareness, and the quality of movement, a different dimension of practice began to emerge. One that emphasized efficiency over effort, awareness over force, and integration over isolated performance.

This shift was not based on theory alone. It was reinforced through years of observation, both in my own practice and in working with others. Patterns became evident. The way a person breathes influences how they move. The way they move influences how they feel. The way they feel influences how they think and respond. These relationships are constant, whether acknowledged or not.

The language used in this book draws heavily from Traditional Chinese Medicine and related systems, where concepts such as Qi, meridians, and the Three Treasures provide a framework for understanding these relationships. While some readers may view this terminology as unfamiliar or abstract, it is best approached as a descriptive model. One that attempts to organize complex, interconnected processes into something that can be observed and applied.

At the same time, modern research in physiology and neuroscience continues to validate many of these observations through different languages. The regulation of the nervous system, the role of breath in autonomic balance, and the adaptability of the human organism all point toward the same fundamental principle: the body is not a collection of separate parts, but a coordinated system shaped by interaction and feedback.

This book is not intended to present a single method or fixed philosophy. Rather, it offers a structured way to explore and understand the energetic dimension of human function through both traditional insight and lived experience.

Ultimately, the value of this material is not found in how it is explained, but in how it is practiced. Through consistent attention, small adjustments, and direct experience, what begins as concept gradually becomes something tangible, measurable, and real.

- Jim Moltzan

Part I — Foundations of Life Energy

1. What is Qi, Chi or Ki?

Chi or Qi (pronounced as "chee") translates to mean "breath" in Chinese. Chi is the life energy that all living creatures require in order to exist. Different cultures call this energy, Ki (from Japanese), Gi (Korean) or Prana (Indian). Chi is a type of energy in the human body and circulates within the blood throughout. Chi flows in a specific pattern from the chest down the front of the arms to the fingers. It then travels up the back of the arms to the head. The chi then travels down the back to the feet and back up the front of the body to the chest. It travels through meridians within the body that can be best described as something similar to the electrical lines on a printed circuit board. There are 12 main meridians and 8 extraordinary ones as well. There are points along these meridians that are known as "pressure points" or acupoints for acupressure and acupuncture.

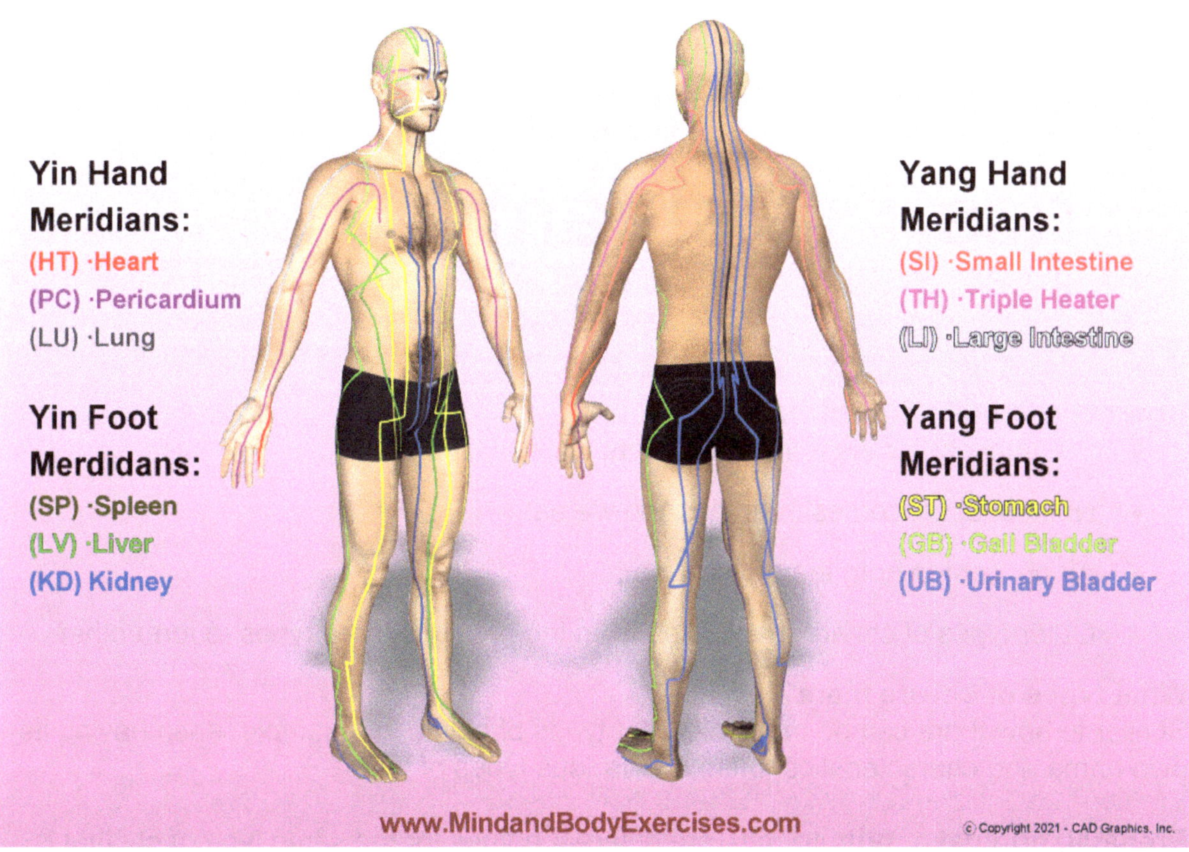

Why is Chi important?
The amount of chi in one's body and the quality of it determines whether an individual is generally healthy or prone to illness. There is a finite amount in our bodies and is gradually exhausted due to age and possible abuses. When it decreases so does the lifespan of the individual.

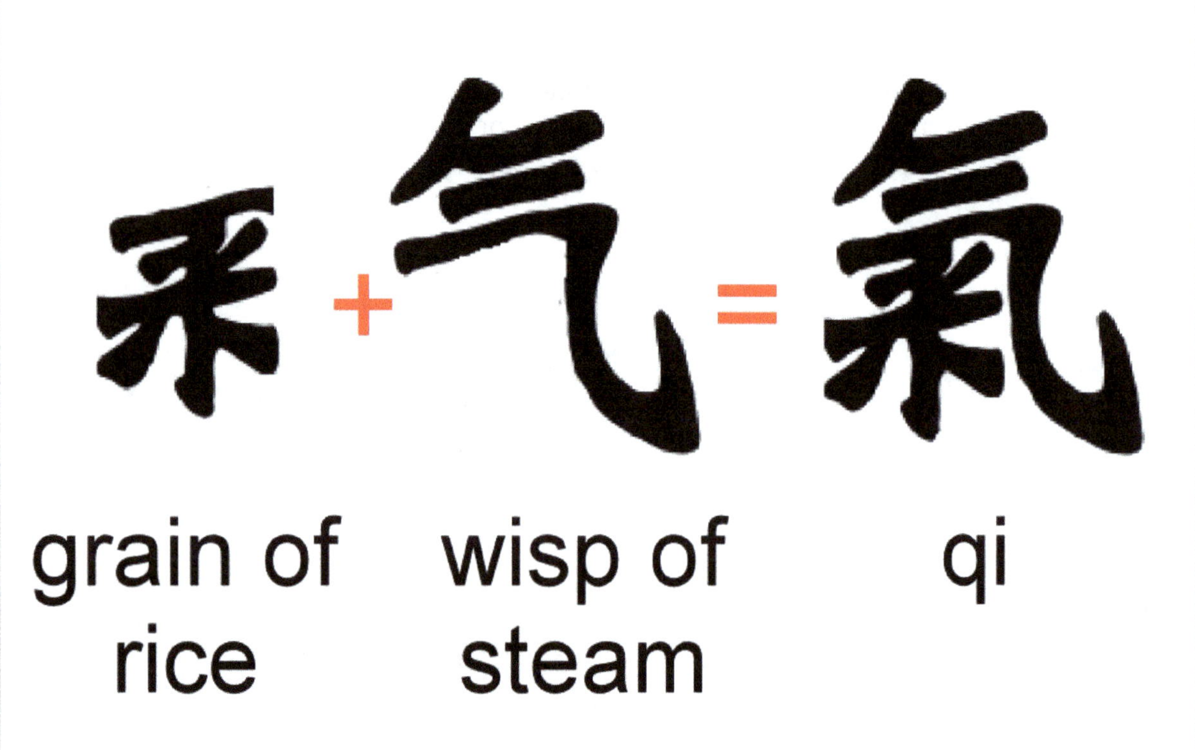

How do we obtain the chi we have?

- Prenatal chi comes from our parents.
- Nutritional chi comes from the food we eat.
- Air chi comes from the air we breathe.
- Other types of chi are manifested from the previous three types to form others.

What types of chi are there?
Similar to how there can be many different types of plants for example, each having its own name and characteristics, there are various types of chi.

Prenatal, original or **primary chi**, are different names for the same type of chi that is inherited from the mother (and father) at the time of conception. At birth, the chi resides in and around the kidneys, eventually spreading throughout the rest of the organs and body. In order for prenatal chi to be maintained, food, drink and air are required. Our health and quality of it are directly linked to the quality of these components. Even if someone's prenatal chi is weak, it can still be properly nourished by proper diet, exercise and lifestyle. Postnatal or nutritional chi and is derived from food and life style. Nutritional chi is responsible for producing the blood as well as providing the body with nourishment. Where the chi circulates, the blood will follow. The blood nourishes the chi; it is a synergistic relationship just is yin and yang.

Pectoral or **air chi** is drawn into our lungs from the air we breathe. People lacking stamina are known to be deficient in air chi. It enables the lungs to control respiratory functions and enables the heart to circulate blood, relying upon the arms and legs to circulate chi throughout the body.

Defensive or **guardian chi (Wei Qi)** circulates on the surface of the body, protecting it from outside influences and dangers. Originating from the food we eat, defensive chi is responsible for the operation of the skin's pores, thereby regulating the body's temperature and ability to provide moisture when needed.

Normal chi or **Zangfu Zhi chi**, is that which circulates through the organs.

Jing Luo Zhi chi is that which circulates through the meridians.

How do I keep what I have?

A proper balance of nutrition, exercise and a healthy lifestyle directly affects the quality and abundance of chi. Emotions and their balance or lack thereof affect the quality of an individual's chi. The 7 emotions are Joy, Anger, Sadness, Grief, Pensiveness, Fear, and Fright. Energy (Chi) is regarded as one of the 3 Treasures or essential components of life, with essence (Jing) and spirit (Shen) being the other two. When energy, essence and spirit are in harmony with one another, the person finds himself or herself alert, healthy and vibrant. Or the opposite, if their treasures are imbalance. If this harmonious flow is disrupted, illness occurs.

Can I get more?

- Better quality food or herbs
- Better quality of air we breathe
- Deep breathing exercises such as Qigong
- Other forms of internal martial arts training such as Tai Chi, Hsing Yi or BaguaZhang

What is Chi Kung, Qigong or Gi Gong?

Exercises originating in India and China, for enhancing or "cultivating" chi. The above names reflect different spellings for the same concept. Cultivate is an appropriate word because, as living things require nourishment and nurturing to grow, chi must be nourished and encouraged to develop.

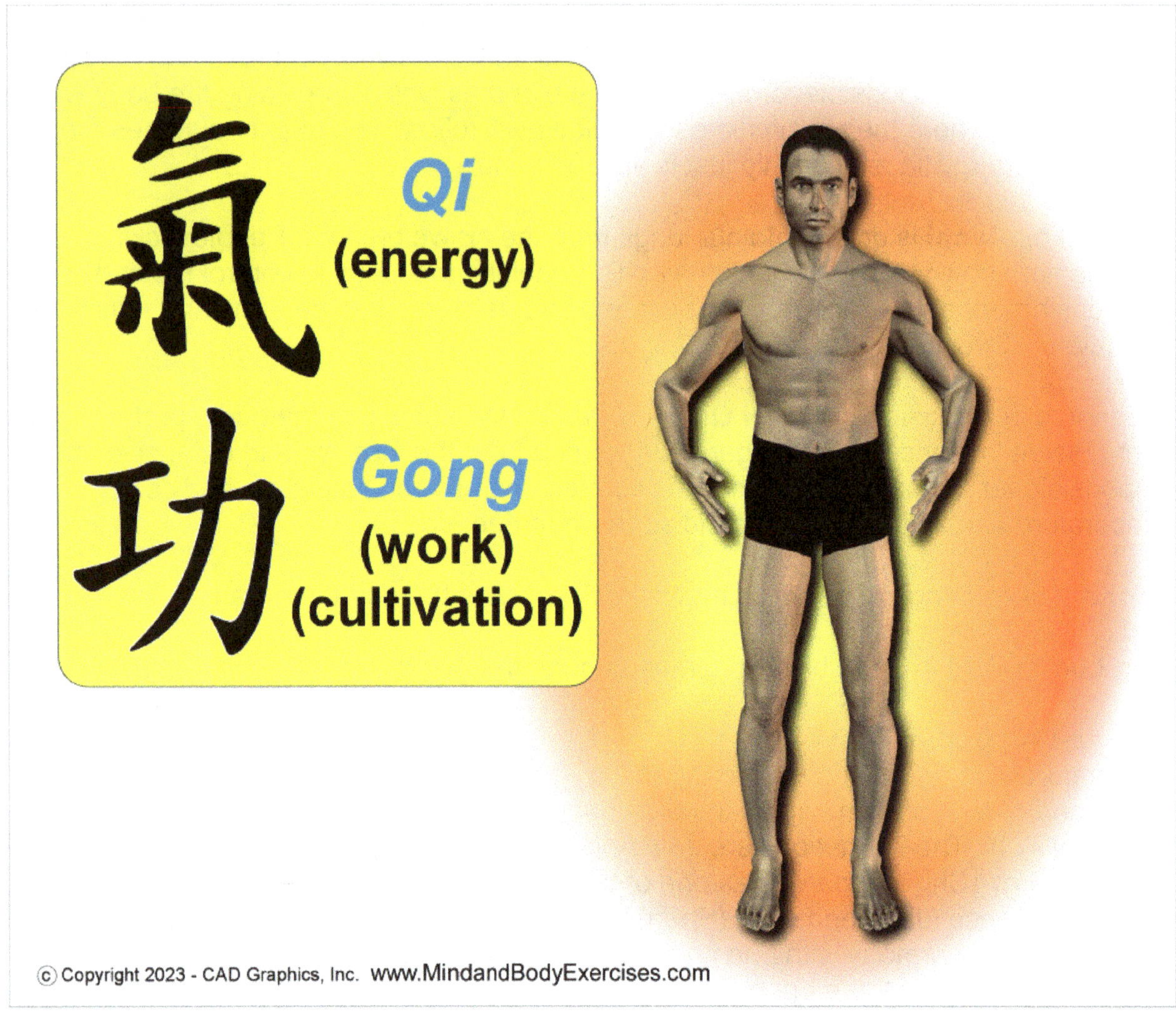

How do these exercises work?
By regulating one's breath and rhythm of it, an individual can begin to affect the parasympathetic nervous system which slows their heart rate, lowers the blood pressure, relieves muscle tension and consequently changes their body chemistry. This is basically the same state of being one achieves while sleeping and is when the body rests, heals and recharges its energy levels.

What are the benefits of practicing these types of exercises?

- Increased energy
- Relief from chronic illnesses
- Increased self-awareness
- Expansion of one's thought process
- Spiritual awareness

- Increased longevity
- Better control of emotions
- Provides a release of one's internal chatter

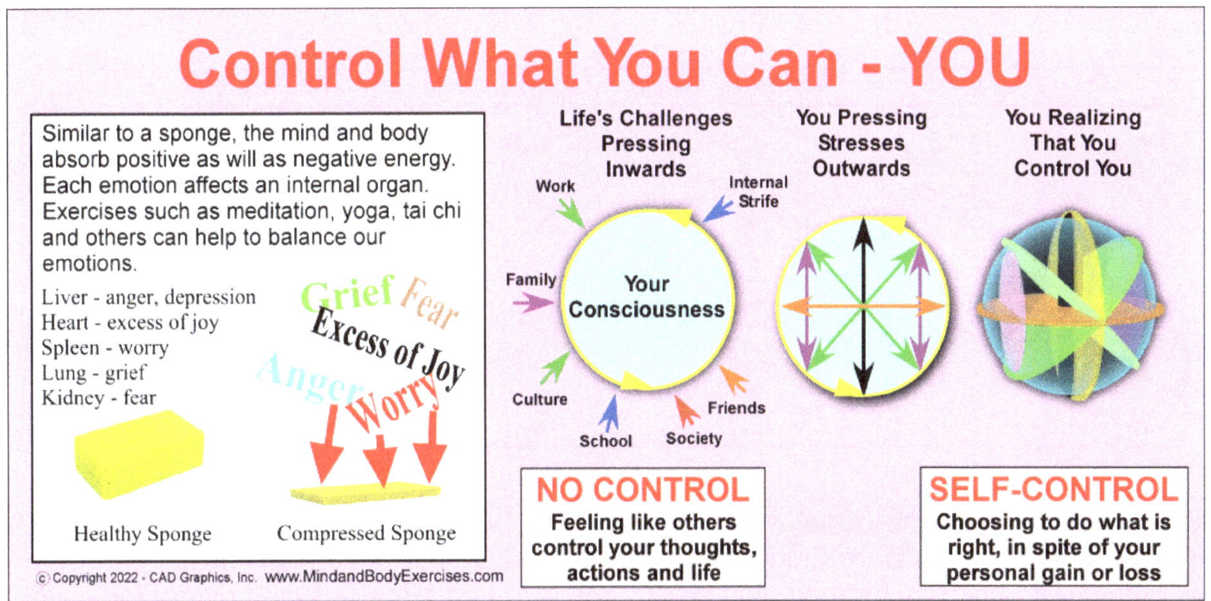

Can Qigong exercises really cure serious diseases and ailments?
It is important to note that the claim of practicing chi kung to overcome illness and promote health is based on countless testimonials of practical cases spanning centuries. If someone is physically impaired, this affects his or her emotions and mental state. Consequently, someone's emotions can easily affect their health, for better or worse. If our psychological and physiological systems function as they should, illness should not occur. Illness occurs when one or more of the body's systems fail in their functions. The specialty of chi kung is to restore and enhance harmonious energy flow, thereby overcoming illness.

What is the difference between Qigong and Nei Dan (Nae Gung)?
Qigong is exercise focusing on increasing one's energy by regulating their breath. Nei Dan is somewhat more advanced in that one uses their thought and awareness to guide and increase their energy throughout the spine and bones within the body.

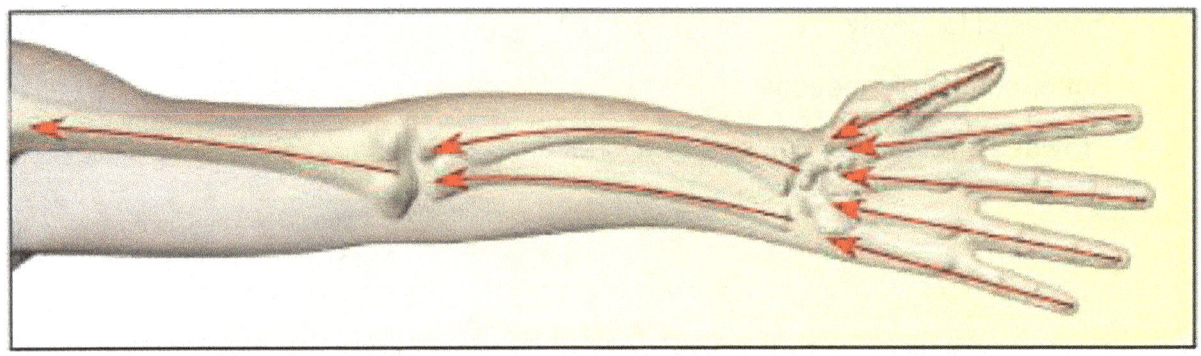

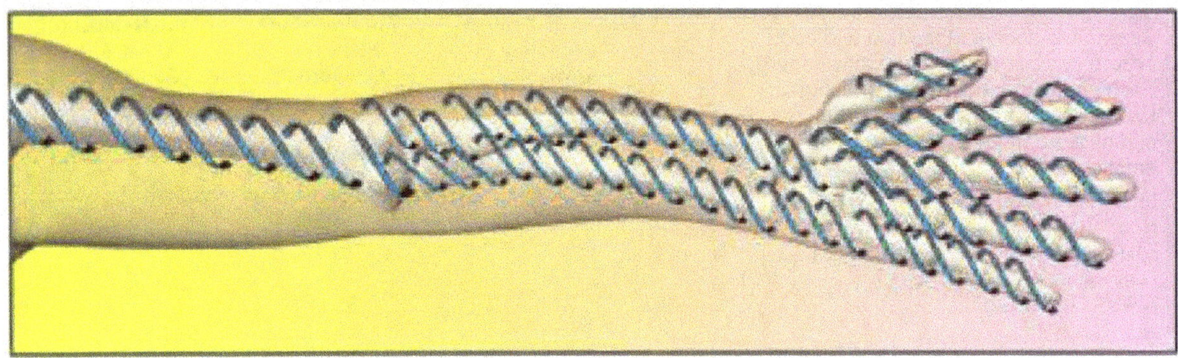

Why pursue these methods?
The American Health Care Crisis might not be as such if all Americans assumed more personal responsibility for their own health. Many spend small fortunes on doctor visits, medication, chiropractic adjustments, massage therapy, acupuncture and other forms of health care and pain relief. Chi kung is relatively cheap to learn, takes little space and only minutes a day to reap the benefits. The only side effects are positive, and it doesn't require a prescription from your doctor.

2. Energy Flow Within the Body

Energy Flow as Organ-to-Organ Transmission: Traditional Chinese Medicine (TCM) teaches that energy or *"Qi"* flows through the body in interconnected organ-to-organ patterns rather than simply circulating from the heart through the bloodstream. This insight reframes how we understand health and movement, emphasizing harmony and balance over mere exertion. This nuanced insight shifts the understanding of physical health from a single focal point to an interconnected system, encouraging movements designed to stimulate this flow comprehensively. This has profound implications for exercise design, rehabilitation, and even stress management, as it integrates bodily systems rather than isolating them.

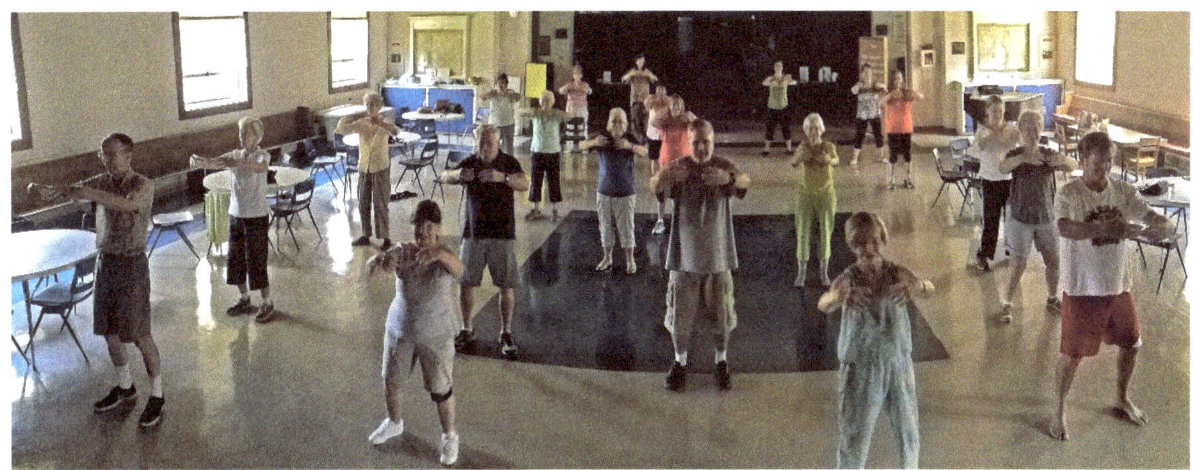

Asymmetry Designed for Functionality: Unlike common exercise patterns that often emphasize symmetrical movement for balance, the asymmetrical nature of these movements mimics biological energy pathways and ensures each part of the body receives appropriate stimulation and energy transfer. This ergonomic approach enhances efficiency and may reduce the chance of injury or overuse affecting one side more than the other.

Breath Control and Relaxation Enable Deeper Energy Work: The synchronized breathing with physical movements, breathing in through the nose, out through the nose or mouth, and coordinating the tongue's position helps extend breath hold times, deepen relaxation, and conserve energy. The concept that tension reduces breath-holding capacity underscores the importance of mental calmness in physical performance and recovery, highlighting a mind-body connection often overlooked in Western fitness paradigms.

Joint Mobility and Energy Flow are Interlinked: The closing set's focus on gently bending and releasing the major joints (shoulders, elbows, wrists, hips, knees, ankles) points to the joints as critical nodes for energy flow, not merely as mechanical hinges. This combined physical and energetic approach maintains joint flexibility and promotes a harmonious rhythm throughout the body, potentially preventing stiffness, spasms, and cramping after exercise.

Energy 'Bank Account' Metaphor Offers Sustainable Health Insight: By likening the body's core energy center to a bank account, the practice teaches the value of replenishing energy rather than depleting it exclusively by movement. This metaphor aligns with modern concepts of energy management, self-care, and sustainability, emphasizing rest and recovery as essential for long-term health benefits, key for athletes, seniors, and anyone seeking balanced vitality.

Cultural Philosophy Enriches Physical Practice: The inclusion of the "Bagua," concept of the figure 8 symbol, at the end of the session introduces a philosophical dimension, uniting physical movement with symbolic meaning. This connection elevates the practice beyond exercise, fostering a deeper sense of continuity, timelessness, and community among participants. It also implies that practice is not just a physical routine but a lifelong commitment to health and awareness.

Longevity and Community Consistency Demonstrate Effectiveness: The fact that this class has been ongoing since 1997 illustrates the adaptability and effectiveness of these principles, as well as the strong community bonds formed among practitioners. The longevity also suggests that such practices can be sustainable and valuable throughout the decades, accommodating newcomers while preserving foundational wisdom. This longevity is a testament to the alignment of tradition with evolving modern health needs.

https://www.youtube.com/watch?v=YU0ulQNZR9M

The video discusses a holistic approach to energy flow in the body, rooted in traditional Chinese medicine and similar philosophies. Unlike typical Western exercise which focuses primarily on cardiovascular activity and the heart, the practice highlighted here emphasizes the flow of energy through a sequence of organs and body parts, following natural patterns rather than symmetrical movements. This method promotes balanced and harmonious movement of energy and blood circulation throughout the body, providing greater overall health benefits.

I guided participants through a closing set of movements designed to relax the major joints of the shoulders, elbows, wrists, hips, knees, ankles, while synchronizing breathing with mindful body awareness. This gradual cool-down process helps prevent muscle cramps and spasms common after mild or intense physical activity by gently bringing energy back to the body's core "battery" or "bank account." The collective movement and breath control encourage relaxation and prolonged breath holding through deliberate tension and release.

This holistic system blends ancient philosophy, breath work, energy theory, and joint mobility into one integrated practice. Rather than isolating fitness goals, it cultivates harmony between body and mind, reflecting the essence of Traditional Chinese Medicine: balanced energy, sustained vitality, and conscious movement.

3. The 3 Treasures

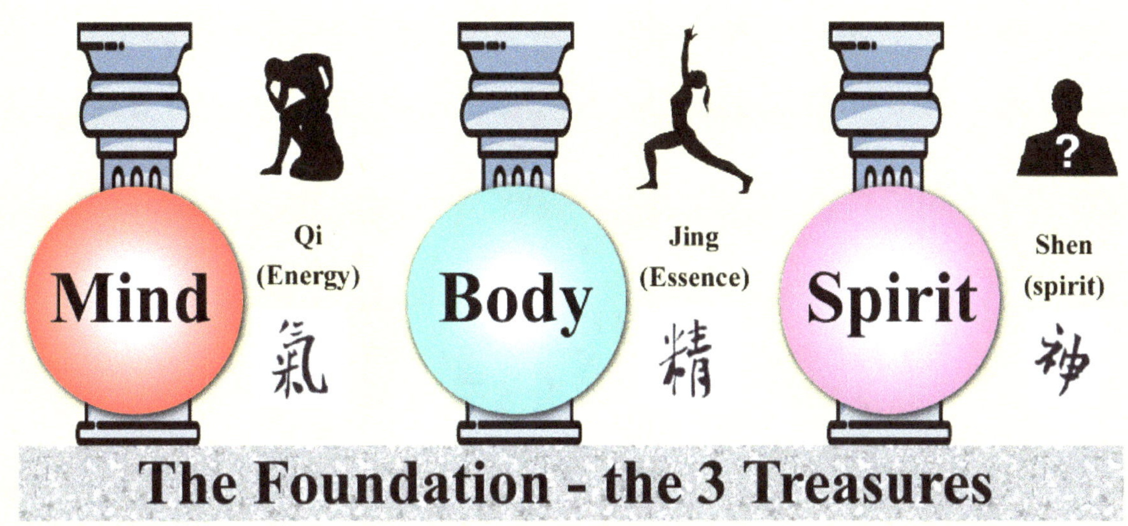

Mind *(Qi)*– How and what you think about and how you process information from sensory input. From the Traditional Chinese Medicine TCM) perspective, the mind is related to the vitality of the breath. Responsible for the blueprint of internal and external functions of the energy force within the body. Qi can be equated to the flame which is the source of the light that illuminates from the candle. The flame eventually consumes the candle. Qi is one's energy or vitality. When Qi is used wisely, one's Jing can last longer. Qi is lost through regular daily activities but gained back through good habits of diet, exercise, breathing, and sleep.

Body *(Jing)* – The physical matter that makes up you and how well it functions. The physical structure of the body's tissue. Responsible for the developmental processes of the body. Jing can be equated to the wick and the wax which is the fuel for the source of the flame. Better quality wax determines the longevity of the candle. One's Jing is determined by genetic inheritance. Jing is depleted over one's lifetime and is not easily replenished.

Spirit *(Shen)* – What you believe as far as beliefs in the unknown, faith, morals, a purpose, etc. The refined level of the mind and higher consciousness. Consists of the spirit, soul, and mind. Responsible for the interaction of destiny & fate. Maintains internal and external functions. Shen can be equated to the light that illuminates a candle. The candle's purpose is to light the darkness. One's Shen is the illumination of their spirit. When one's Jing and Qi are in abundance, Shen is released. Shen is divided further into the mind (shen), the intellect (yi), the corporeal soul (po), willpower (zhi) and the ethereal soul (hun). These 5 shen are a topic for another discussion.

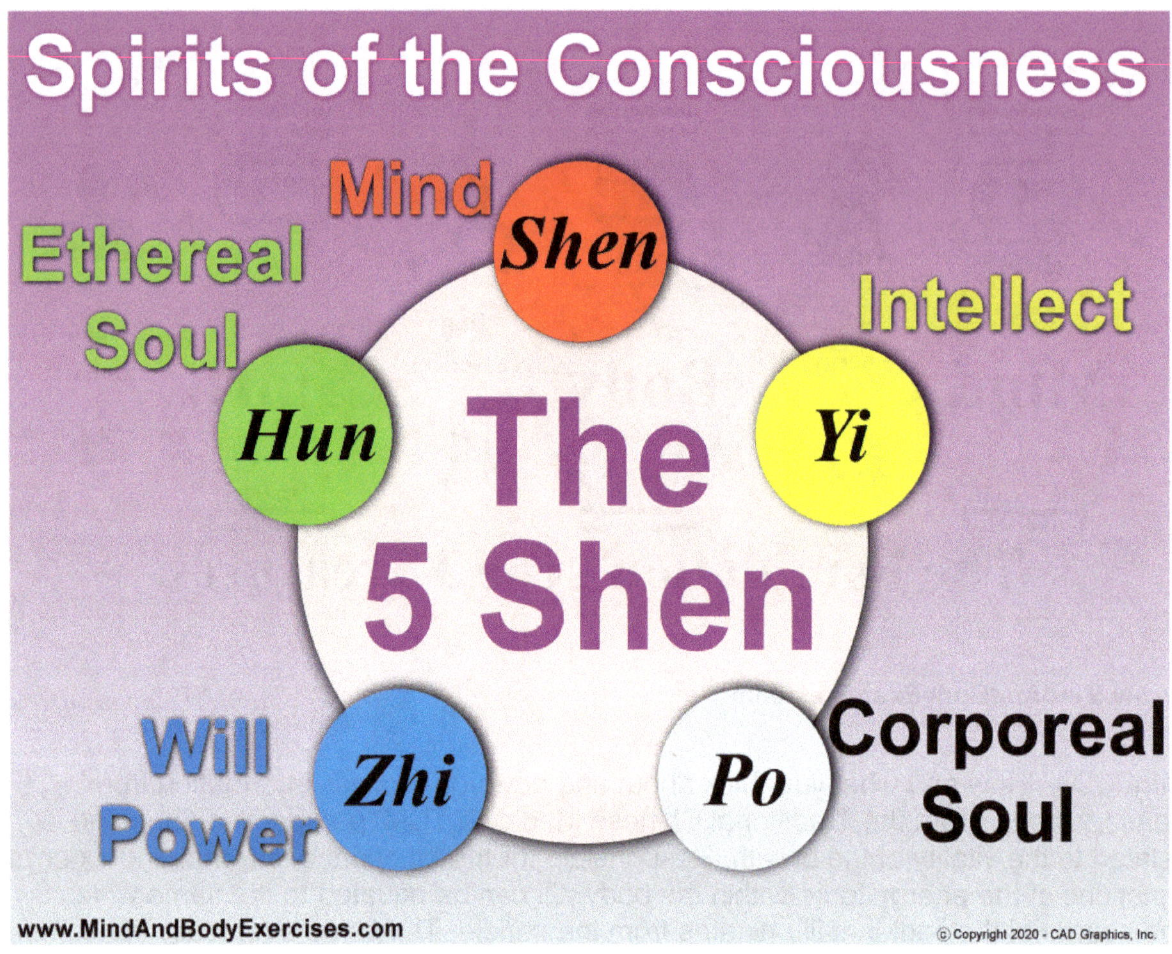

These three treasures are the most valuable things that we all possess. Without these 3, we have no family, no friends, no career, no big house, no internet. What we sometimes see today as "new" is indeed rather old. This concept of the 3 Treasures comes from Taoism, a philosophy that is over 2000 years old, originating around 500 BCE. These are universal truths that are hard to debate. We all need to take care of our own "treasures" before we can be of benefit to those around us. Breathe deeper, exercise more, eat better, and earn a good night's sleep by being active and relieving stress during the day.

Modern science and research seek to label and dissect any and all things, intending to assign a name or label to all that *is* and sometimes that which *is not*. With this realization, we can see from the graphic below the many sub-categories that are now thought to be parts of the original concept of mind, body, and spirit.

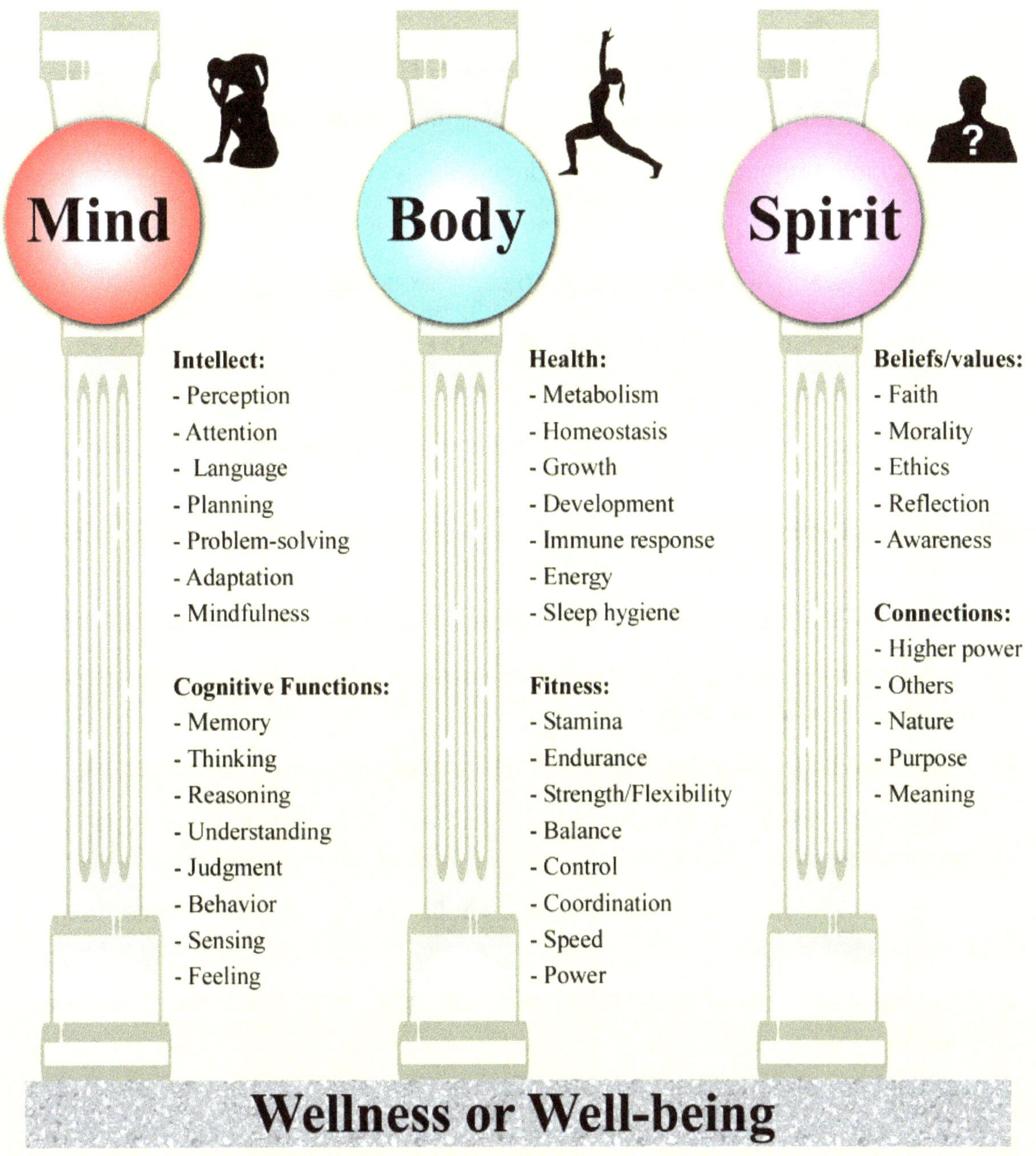

www.MindAndBodyExercises.com

The mind is comprised of various components:
Intellect:

- Perception – recognizing and acknowledging sensory stimuli.
- Attention – ability to focus on specific thoughts and stimuli.
- Language – understanding and producing speech and writing.
- Planning – ability to formulate a strategy or process.
- Problem-solving – finding solutions to complex issues.
- Decision-making – making choices among options.
- Adaptation – being able to change and adjust thoughts, feelings, and actions.
- Mindfulness – an awareness of current thoughts, feelings, and surroundings.

Cognitive Functions:

- Memory – storage and retrieval of information.
- Thinking – the mental process of considering or reasoning about something.
- Reasoning – the process of drawing conclusions or making inferences based on evidence and logical principles.
- Understanding – to comprehend the meaning or significance of something.
- Judgment – the ability to make considered decisions or come to sensible conclusions.
- Behavior – the actions or reactions of an individual in response to external or internal stimuli.
- Sensing – the process of detecting and responding to stimuli through the sensory organs.
- Feelings – experiences of emotions.

The body can be broken down into various categories:
Health:

- Metabolism – chemical processes that occur within living organisms.
- Homeostasis – the body's ability to manage and regulate stable internal bodily functions and conditions.
- Growth/development – physical changes throughout a living organism's lifespan.
- Immune response – ability of the body to defend against pathogens.
- Energy – the amount of physical power that can be drawn upon.

- Sleep hygiene – the quality of an individual's ability to rest and recover.

Fitness:

- Survival – on the most basic level, the ability to stay alive.
- Stamina – ability to sustain prolonged physical for an extended time without fatigue.
- Endurance – the muscular system's capacity to sustain activity.
- Strength – the ability of muscles to exert force against resistance
- Flexibility – the range of motion available at a joint or group of joints
- Balance – the ability to maintain the body's position, whether stationary or while moving.
- Control – to manage and direct the body's movements precisely and efficiently.
- Coordination – ability to use different parts of the body together smoothly and efficiently.
- Speed – to move quickly across the ground or move limbs rapidly for a specific purpose.
- Power – ability to exert maximum force in the shortest amount of time.

Spirit can be interpreted through numerous facets:
Beliefs/values:

- Faith – belief in principles of an organized religion or spiritual practice.
- Morality – the ability to differentiate between what is considered right and wrong.
- Ethics – a system of moral principles.
- Reflection – the ability to be aware of one's own thoughts and actions.
- Awareness – a sense of one's self, surroundings, and relative environment.

Connections:

- Higher power – a sense of a greater presence beyond themselves.
- Others – relationships with people, and community.
- Nature – relationships with all living creatures and the environment.
- Purpose – a reason to wake up every day.
- Meaning – realization of one's reason for existing

4. Three Treasures plus Emptiness

In Taoist cultivation theory, the "Three Treasures" (*sān bǎo*) of *jīng, qì* and *shén* describe successive refinements of being: from bodily substance to energy to spirit. Alongside and underpinning this transformative process is the principle of *xū*, often translated "emptiness", "void", or "hollow openness". Xū is not mere nothingness, but a dynamic receptive ground that allows emergence, transformation, and return. This essay explicates the meaning of xū, its relation to the Three Treasures, and how classical Taoist texts articulate this interplay.

The Three Treasures: Jīng, Qì and Shén
The Three Treasures are central in Taoist internal alchemy (*nèi dān*) as the raw materials and vehicles of transformation.

Treasure	Chinese	Key meaning	Role in cultivation
Essence	精 (*jīng*)	The dense, material-vital substance (including inherited vitality, reproductive substance) (Bartek, 2024)	Reserved, refined and conserved; the "root" of life and alchemical process.
Vital energy / breath	氣 (*qì*)	The dynamic life-force, movement, breath, transformation of substance into energy (Bartek, 2024)	Circulates, refines essence into spirit; bridges body and spirit.
Spirit / consciousness	神 (*shén*)	The refined, luminous aspect of awareness, spirit, mind, divine seed (Pregadio, 2009)	The outcome of refinement; the luminous presence and the vehicle of transcendence.

In internal-alchemy texts such as the Wuzhen Pian attributed to Zhang Boduan, the Three Treasures are explicitly cited as the ingredients of the internal elixir:

"...the body contains the essential components: these Three Treasures are jīng, qì and shén."

Thus, the alchemist's work is to refine jīng → qì → shén and finally to integrate with the Way (道).

The Concept of Xū

Definition and nuance
The Chinese character 虚 (*xū*) conveys "emptiness", "voidness", "hollowness", "open space", "vacancy", but importantly also "receptivity", "openness", "ungrasped potential". In Taoist texts, xū is often the invisible space or still ground that allows form, movement, being, and return.

For example, in the classic Tao Te Ching by Laozi, Chapter 11 states:

"Thirty spokes join at one hub; it is the emptiness (xū) that makes the wagon useful. Cast clay into a vessel; it is the emptiness inside that makes it useful. Cut out doors and windows to make a room; it is the emptiness within that makes it inhabitable." (Tao Te Ching by Lao Tzu – Verse 11 – Three Translations, 2021)

And Chapter 16:

*"Attain complete emptiness (xū); hold fast to stillness. The myriad beings arise - yet each returns to its root." (*Tao Te Ching by Lao Tzu – Verse 11 – Three Translations, 2021)

Thus xū is both origin and destination. It is the silent ground from which being arises and to which it returns.

Xū in internal alchemy
In internal alchemy (nèi dān), xū becomes the "vessel" or "cauldron" within the practitioner, as an inner space, body-mind field of openness, into which essence, energy and spirit are guided. According to scholarship:

> *"In meditative practices, they visualize the human body as a cauldron that refines the internal vital forces including essence (jīng), pneuma (qì), and spirit (shén) to produce an internal elixir…"* (Wuzhen Pian 悟真篇 Also Known as "Essay on the [Immediate] Awakening to Truth", "Chapters on Awakening to Perfection" - UBC Library Open Collections, n.d.)

Also:
"It regards humans as a set of tripods and stoves for refining and enhancing one's own life energy (jīng, qì, shén) … The first stage involves replenishing jīng, qì and shén, … the final is returning to emptiness." (Golden Elixir Press, n.d.)

Hence, xū is the operative "space" in which the refinement jīng → qì → shén occurs, and into which shén finally dissolves.

Relationship of Xū to the Three Treasures

Here is how xū operates at each stage of the alchemical process:

Transformation stage	Role of Xū	Implication for cultivation
jīng → qì	The practitioner first quiets distractions, reserves essence, cultivates stillness—creating an inner emptiness (xū) so that jīng does not scatter.	Cultivating "emptied receptivity": less sensory input, fewer desires, conserving jīng.
qì → shén	Energy (qì) flows within the "empty vessel" (xū), unimpeded by conceptual/motional turbulence; this allows qì to transform into shén.	Cultivation shifts to subtle awareness, opening to spirit, refining vital energy in the void.
shén → Return to Xū	At completion, the refined shén merges into emptiness (xū), dissolving the individual self into universal ground (道). The Three Treasures originate from xū and return to xū.	The goal: abiding in xū as "Spirit and Emptiness united as one".

In other words:
xū is neither an added "fourth treasure" nor merely an absence, but the field of transformation and integration of the Three Treasures. Without xū: jīng stagnates, qì scatters, shén remains bound. With xū: alchemy is possible, transformation flows, transcendence becomes attainable.

Classical Source Quotations

Here are selected quotations with Chinese original and annotated translation:

1. From Tao Te Ching, Ch. 11
    - *"Thirty spokes join at one hub; yet it is the emptiness therein that gives the wheel its use. Kneading clay to form a vessel; yet it is the emptiness therein that makes the vessel useful…"* (Dao De Jing [Tao Te Ching], by Lao Zi [Lao Tzu] in Side-by-Side Translation: Chapter 11, n.d.)

2. From Tao Te Ching, Ch. 16
    - *"Attain complete emptiness; hold fast to stillness. The myriad beings all arise - I watch their return. The myriad things flourish and each returns to its root. Returning to the root is called stillness. Stillness is called returning to destiny. Returning to destiny is called the Constant. Knowing the Constant is called clarity…"* (Garofalo, n.d.)

3. From Wuzhen Pian

- Though specific lines are metaphorical and sparse, one commentary notes: *"The body contains the essential components. These Three Treasures are jīng, qì and shén."* (Wikipedia contributors, 2025)
- And that this text visualizes the human body as a cauldron refining the Three Treasures. (Wuzhen Pian 悟真篇 Also Known as "Essay on the [Immediate] Awakening to Truth", "Chapters on Awakening to Perfection" - UBC Library Open Collections, n.d.)

4. Scholarly exegesis: *"The first stage involves replenishing essence, breath and spirit … and the final is returning to emptiness."* (Golden Elixir Press, n.d.)
5. Interpretation of the Three Treasures in Chinese culture: *"The ancient Daoists believed that man exists inseparably between heaven and earth and that there is a mutual relationship between these three (heaven, earth, man) …"* in relation to jīng, qì, shén. (Bartek, 2024)

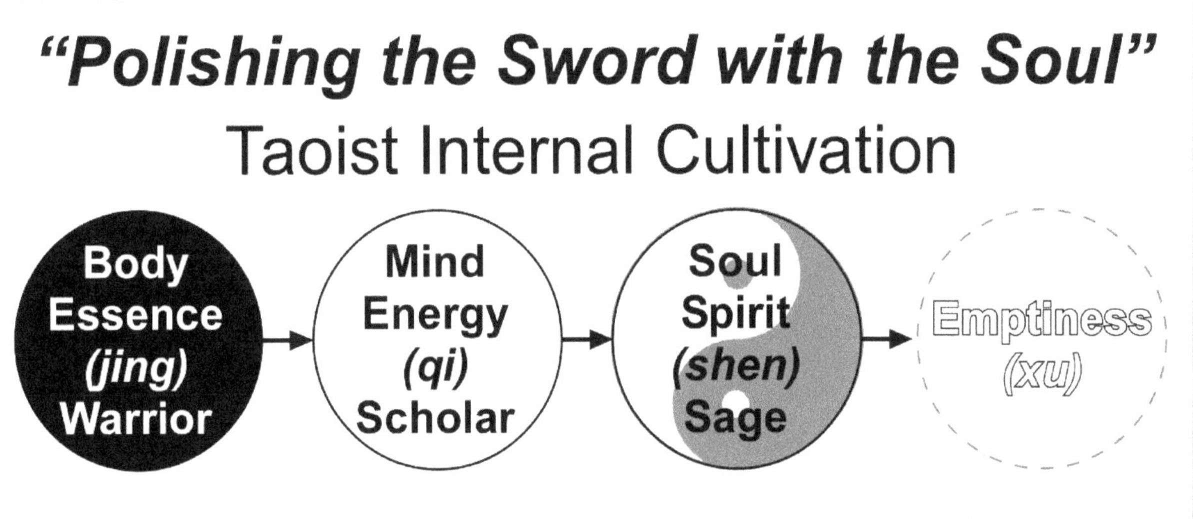

Summary

- The Three Treasures (jīng, qì, shén) chart an inner alchemical journey: the body's essence → refined energy → luminous spirit.
- Xū (emptiness) is not a fourth treasure but the primordial field within which the alchemical transformation occurs and to which it ultimately returns.
- Cultivation involves first creating receptivity and emptiness (xū) to conserve essence, then refining energy in the vessel of emptiness, and finally abiding in emptiness as spirit dissolves into the Way.
- The classical Taoist tradition (via Laozi's Tao Te Ching and texts like Wuzhen Pian) illustrates this with metaphors of wheel hubs, vessels, cauldrons, and return to root.

- Practically, meditation and Qigong aim to "clear the vessel", "quiet the hub", "walk the empty path" so that the Three Treasures can operate in harmony.

References

Bartek. (2024, June 28). *Jing, Qi, Shen – Die drei Schätze*. Path of Dao. https://path-of-dao-qigong.ch/en/jing-qi-shen/

Dao De Jing [Tao Te ching], by Lao Zi [Lao Tzu] in Side-by-Side Translation: Chapter 11. (n.d.). YellowBridge. https://www.yellowbridge.com/onlinelit/daodejing11.php?utm_source=chatgpt.com

Garofalo, M. P. (n.d.). *Dao de Jing, Laozi, Chapter 16*. https://mpgtaijiquan.blogspot.com/2015/05/dao-de-jing-laozi-chapter-16.html?utm_source=chatgpt.com

Golden Elixir Press. (n.d.). *Foundations of Internal Alchemy — A slideshow*. Scribd. https://www.scribd.com/document/99535352/Foundations-of-Internal-Alchemy-A-Slideshow?utm_source=chatgpt.com

Pregadio, F. (2009). Awakening to Reality: The "Regulated Verses" of the Wuzhen pian, a Taoist Classic of Internal Alchemy. In *Golden Elixir Press*. https://www.goldenelixir.com/files/Introduction_to_Awakening_to_Reality.pdf?utm_source=chatgpt.com

The Project Gutenberg eBook of *Dao de Jing*, by Lao Zi. (n.d.). https://www.gutenberg.org/files/49965/49965-h/49965-h.htm?utm_source=chatgpt.com

Tao Te Ching by Lao Tzu – Verse 11 – Three translations. (2021, November 30). Vishy's Blog. https://vishytheknight.wordpress.com/2021/11/30/tao-te-ching-by-lao-tzu-verse-11-three-translations/?utm_source=chatgpt.com

Wikipedia contributors. (2025, October 1). Wuzhen pian. Wikipedia. https://en.wikipedia.org/wiki/Wuzhen_pian?utm_source=chatgpt.com

Wuzhen pian 悟真篇 also known as "Essay on the [Immediate] Awakening to Truth", "Chapters on Awakening to Perfection" - UBC Library Open Collections. (n.d.). https://open.library.ubc.ca/cIRcle/collections/ubccommunityandpartnerspublicati/52387/items/1.0416054?utm_source=chatgpt.com

5. Four-Phase Expansion of the Jing–Qi–Shen Developmental Model

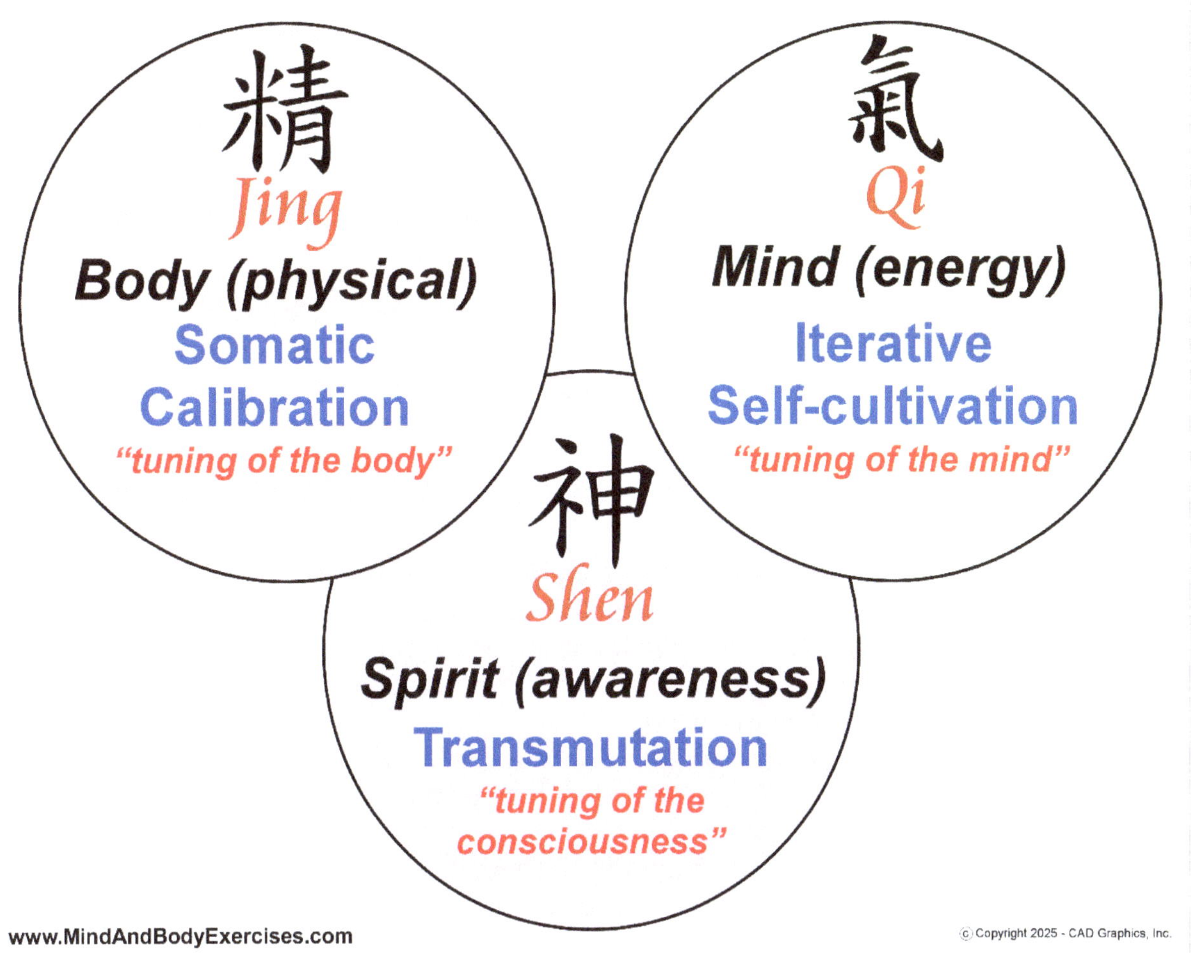

Phase 1 — Foundational Awareness: Somatic Calibration (Jing)
Phase 1 represents the foundational stage where the practitioner learns to attune their physical body, **the *Jing* level,** through heightened somatic awareness and physiological regulation. At this level, the focus is on:

- **Interoception:** sensing internal signals such as breath, heartbeat, and muscular tension
- **Proprioception:** detecting body position and micro-adjustments
- **Regulatory Responsiveness:** adjusting posture, breathing, and alignment

Somatic calibration stabilizes the "*base material*" of the human system. In Taoist internal arts, this is the earliest refinement of Jing: raw essence becoming cleaner, clearer, and more governable.

Neuroscientifically, this phase strengthens communication between the insula (interoceptive awareness), anterior cingulate cortex (attention and motivation), and prefrontal cortex (regulation and decision-making). When these systems integrate, the practitioner becomes capable of sensing imbalances long before they erupt into dysfunction (Khalsa et al., 2018).

This phase is therefore concerned with:

- Cultivating *"felt sense"*
- Stabilizing the nervous system
- Learning to *"hear"* the body
- Establishing physical coherence

Without Phase 1, progression into deeper phases becomes imbalanced or potentially unsafe.

This is the **Jing → stability** transformation.

Phase 2 — Cyclical Refinement: Iterative Self-cultivation (Qi)
Once somatic clarity is established, the practitioner advances toward the mental-energetic domain, **the *Qi* level**. This phase introduces iterative practice and self-correction, forming the living engine of personal development.
Here, the operating principle is **iteration**:

Practice → feedback → correction → integration → renewed practice

Across martial arts, meditation, and qigong lineages, this cyclical refinement is recognized as **gongfu (kung fu),** not mere skill, but the cultivated discipline earned through dedicated repetition. Each iteration reshapes:

- Motor pathways
- Emotional patterns
- Cognitive habits
- Energetic circulation

Modern neuroscience parallels this with **experience-dependent neuroplasticity** or the gradual restructuring of brain networks for resilience, emotional regulation, and attentional stability (Davidson & McEwen, 2012).

Spiritually and philosophically, Phase 2 is where one begins forging ***de*** (virtue, cultivated inner power). The practitioner transitions from merely *feeling* the body to *shaping* the self.

At this stage, Qi becomes more coherent and directed. Mental habits are tuned, intentions sharpen, and discipline becomes embodied.

This is the **Qi → refinement** transformation.

Phase 3 — Synthetic Integration: Transmutation (Shen)
Phase 3 transitions from refinement into **whole-system synthesis**, corresponding to the ***Shen* level,** with awareness, meaning, and inner illumination.

Here the practitioner no longer simply adjusts the body (Phase 1) or trains the mind through iteration (Phase 2). Instead, they **convert base tendencies into higher capacities**. This includes:

- fear → insight
- pain → empathy
- discipline → wisdom
- adversity → meaning

This is the essence of **transmutation** in internal alchemy (neidan):

Jing → Qi → Shen → back to emptiness and clarity

Physiologically, this level parallels harmonization of endocrine rhythms, autonomic coherence, and emotional centers that once produced reactivity but now produce calm presence.
Psychologically, the practitioner embodies authenticity rather than performance. Their presence becomes stabilizing to others, as they can become "the light that guides."
Phase 3 is where:

- the body listens
- the mind learns
- *consciousness reorients* toward clarity

This is the **Shen → illumination** transformation.

Bring it all together - the Harmonization (Integration of Jing–Qi–Shen)
My diagrams and progression of images naturally imply a fourth phase, which is the integrative stage where Jing, Qi, and Shen no longer operate as separate domains but revolve in a recursive living spiral.
Here, the practitioner reaches a point where:

- Somatic calibration is continuous and automatic
- Iterative self-cultivation is self-initiating
- Transmutation becomes a way of life

- All three influence each other simultaneously

This is the phase where the *circle completes itself yet continues upward,* a spiral path rather than a linear one.

In this 4th Phase the practitioner embodies:

1. **Physical alignment (Jing)**
   Effortless posture, efficient movement, regulated physiology.

2. **Mental clarity and energetic coherence (Qi)**
   Stable attention, balanced emotions, refined intentions.

3. **Spiritual awareness (Shen)**
   Insight, compassion, spaciousness, wisdom.

4. **Harmonized integration**
   The practitioner is no longer "performing techniques" as
   they have become the technique.

This is the lived outcome of the entire model of the *Warrior, Scholar* and *Sage*:

Somatic Calibration → Iterative Self-cultivation → Transmutation → Integrated Being.

How the Four Phases Correspond to my Diagrams (Stages 1–4)

Stage 1 (Jing/Qi/Shen circles):
Introduces the classical triad, three aspects as separate yet related.

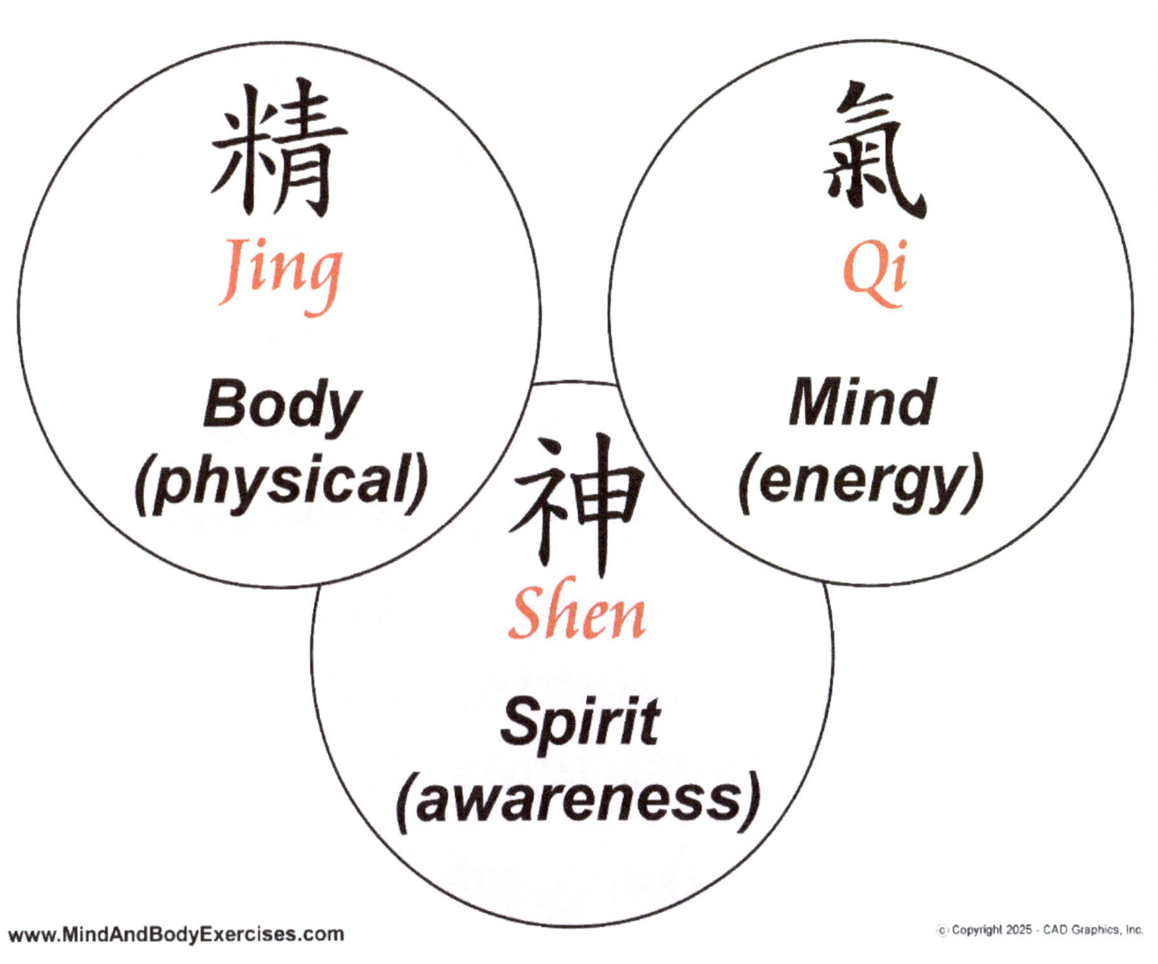

Stage 2 (Physiology/Psychology/Philosophy overlay):
Connects each classical aspect with modern disciplines.

This becomes the foundation of Phase 1.

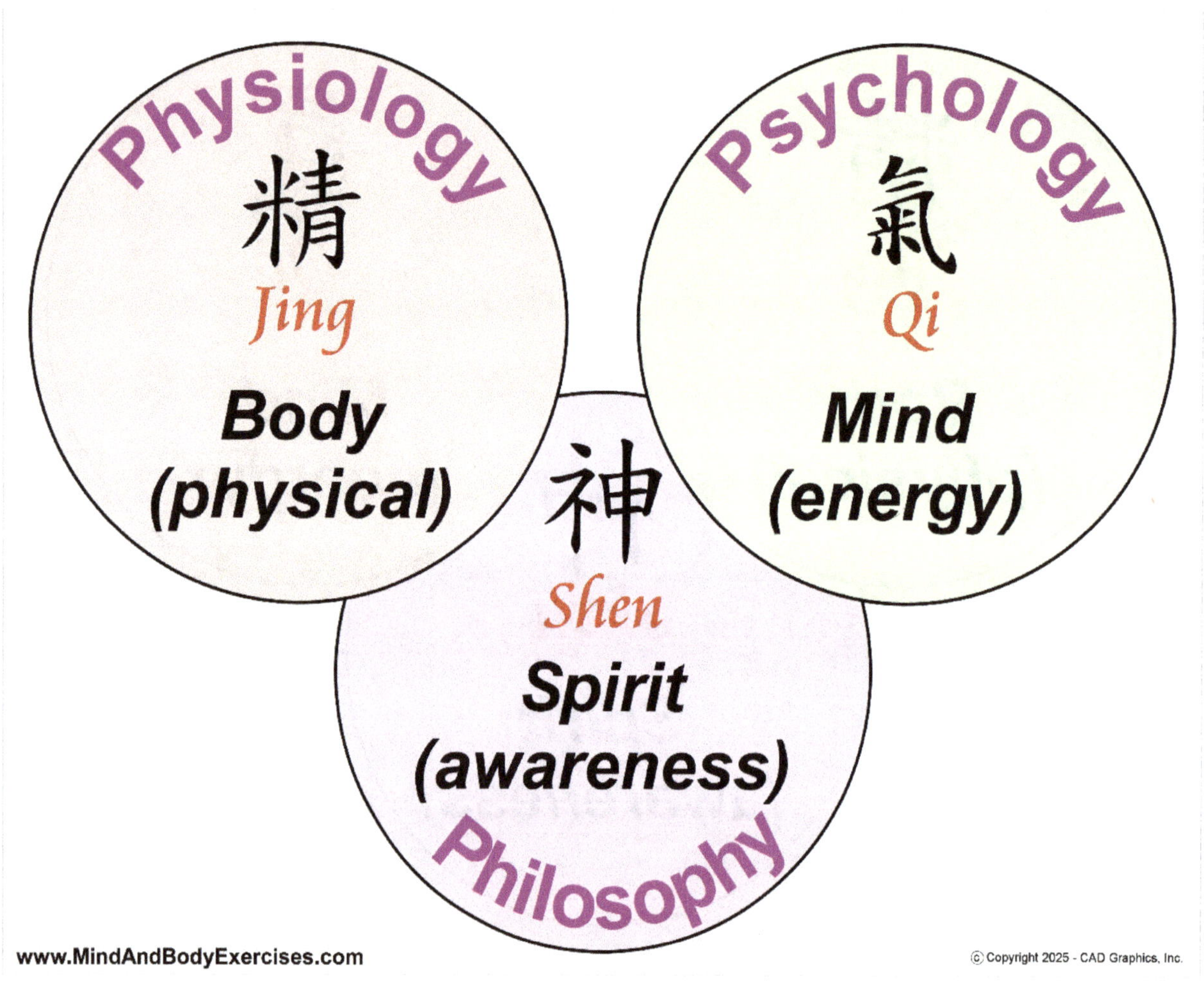

Stage 3 (Somatic Calibration / Iterative Self-cultivation / Transmutation overlay): Maps each classical component into the three functional processes.

This is Phase 2 and Phase 3.

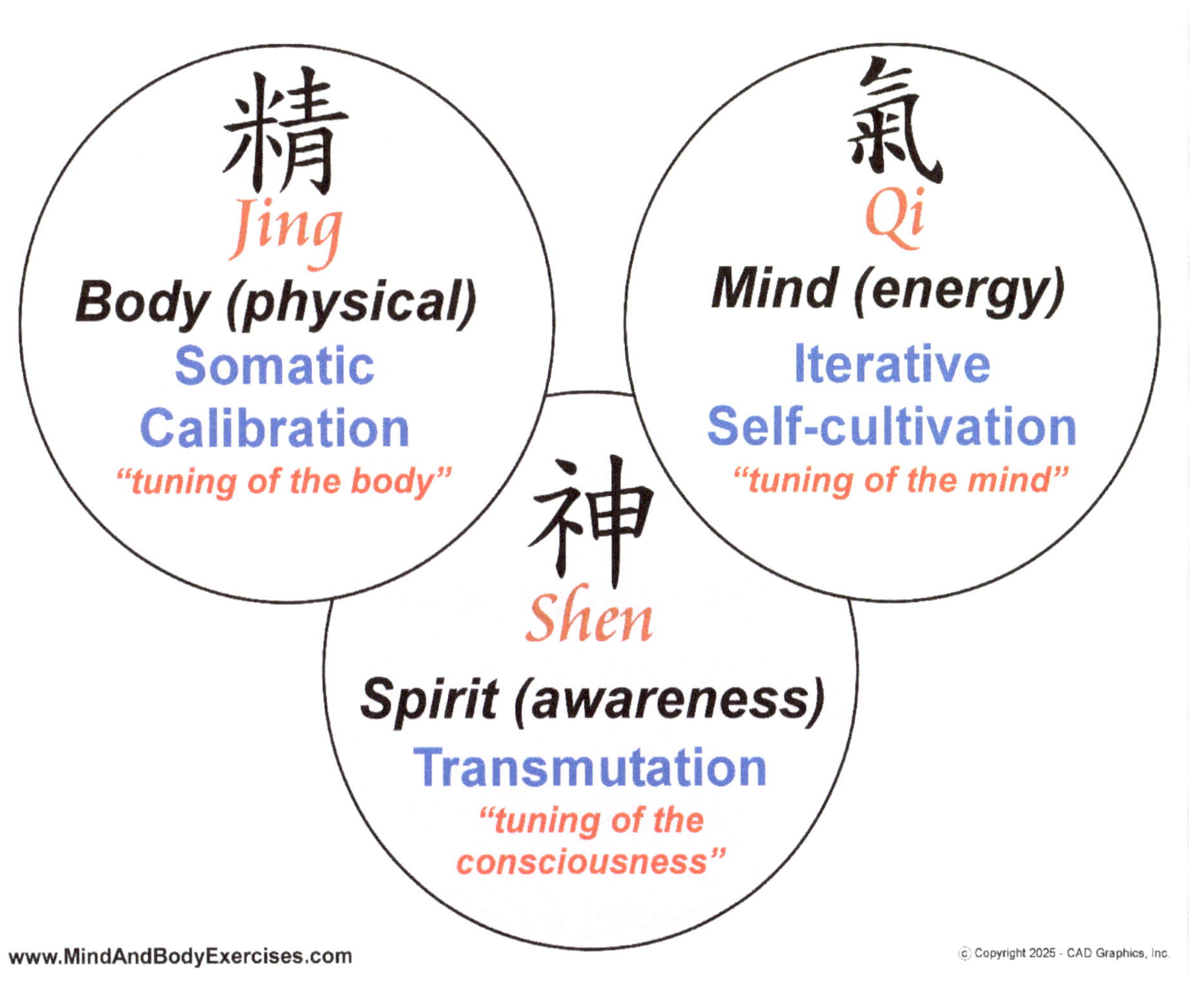

Stage 4 (Full elaborated diagram with figures):
Demonstrates the mature, embodied expression of all three components working in harmony.

This represents Phase 4.

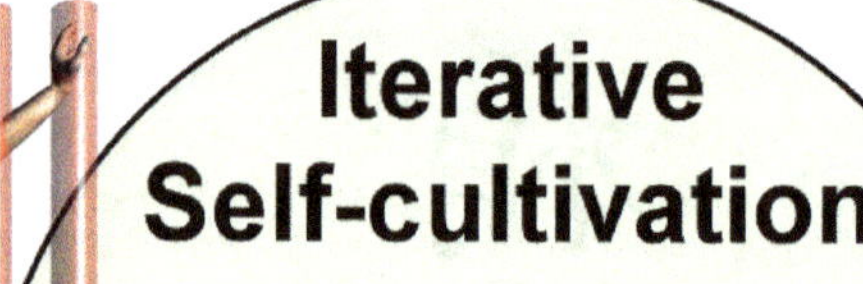

Somatic Calibration

refines awareness and alignment

"tuning of the body"

Somatic Awareness (interoception)
consciously perceiving sensations of tension, breath, heartbeat, and alignment

Interoceptive Accuracy (cognitive processes)
the brain's interpretation of internal bodily cues

Regulatory Responsiveness (adjustments)
the capacity to modify one's physiological state, through breathing, posture, or focus to achieve balance

Iterative Self-cultivation

builds discipline and stability

"tuning of the mind"

mindful practice, reflection, and correction

the ongoing cycle of practice - feedback - adjustment - integration.

deliberate repetition that rewires synaptic pathways for stability, emotional regulation, and self-mastery

Each repetition deepens skill while gradually refining the character, much like tempering a sword through alternating heat and cooling.

Transmutation

realizes integration and illumination

"tuning of the consciousness"

the conversion of base tendencies into higher expression

Through calibrated awareness and continuous self-cultivation, internal friction and limitation become fuel for illumination

Regular engagement in mindful movement or performance retrains the nervous system to operate in coherence, balancing sympathetic activation (energy, readiness) and parasympathetic recovery (calm, restoration).

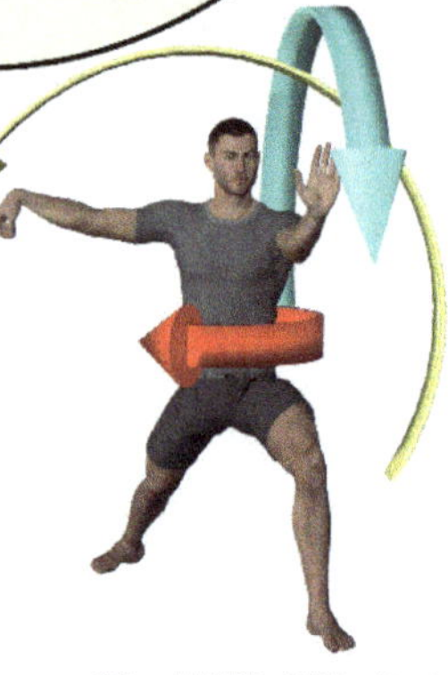

www.MindAndBodyExercises.com

Integrated Summary

- **Phase 1—Somatic Calibration:** tuning the body (Jing), establishing stability and awareness.
- **Phase 2—Iterative Self-cultivation:** tuning the mind (Qi), cultivating discipline, neuroplasticity, and virtuous habits.
- **Phase 3—Transmutation:** tuning the consciousness (Shen), converting tendencies into illumination.
- **Phase 4—Recursive Harmonization:** integrating Jing–Qi–Shen into a coherent, unified mode of being.

Together these phases describe a **complete developmental alchemical model** bridging Taoist tradition, neuroscience, psychology, and embodied martial philosophy.

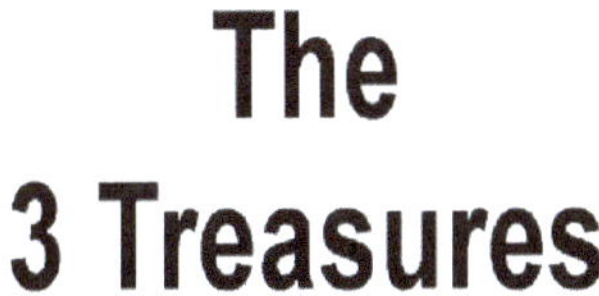

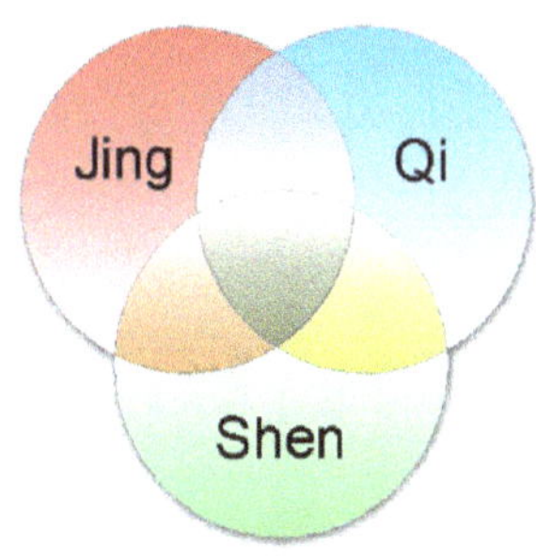

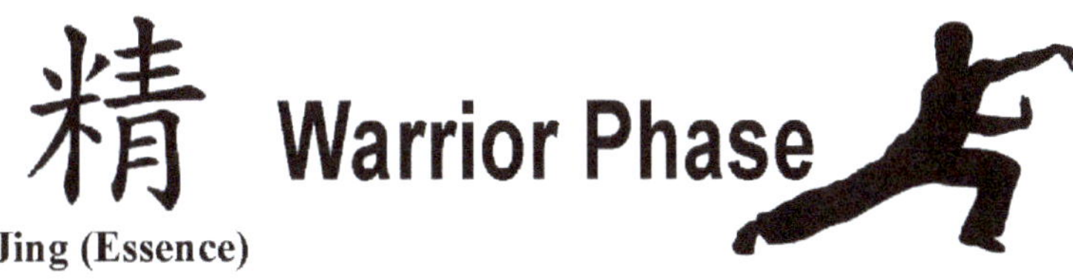

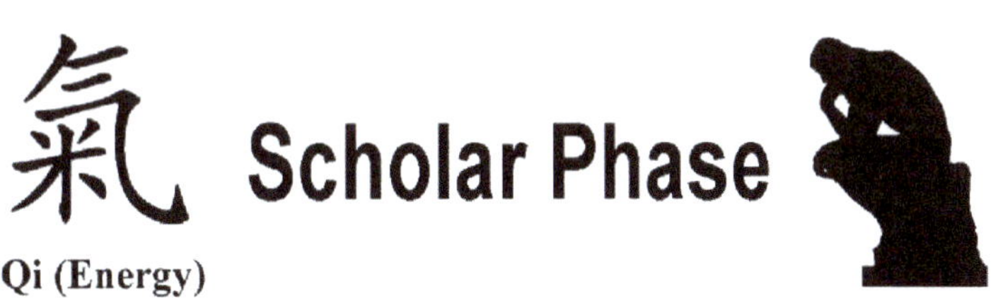

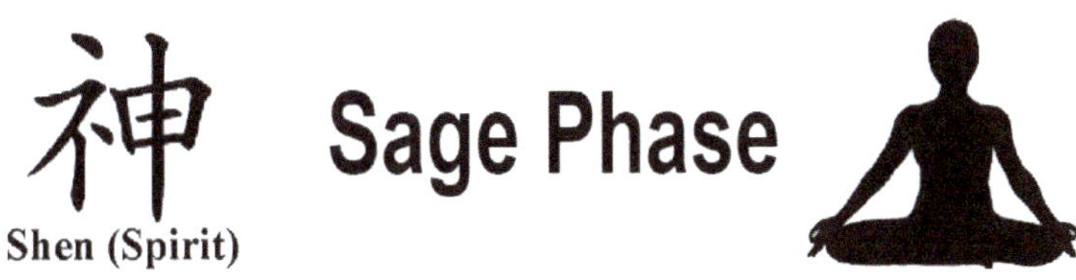

Part II — Meridian Systems and Energetic Anatomy

6. 12 Meridians vs. 8 Extraordinary Vessels

Understanding the Difference Between the 12 Primary Meridians and the 8 Extraordinary Vessels in Traditional Chinese Medicine

Traditional Chinese Medicine (TCM) views the human body as an intricate network of energy channels that govern physical, emotional, and spiritual health. Two key components of this system are the **12 Primary Meridians** and the **8 Extraordinary Vessels**. Though they are interconnected, they serve distinctly different roles in maintaining balance and vitality. Understanding this distinction provides deeper insight into how TCM approaches healing, longevity, and self-cultivation (Maciocia, 2005).

The 12 Primary Energy Meridians

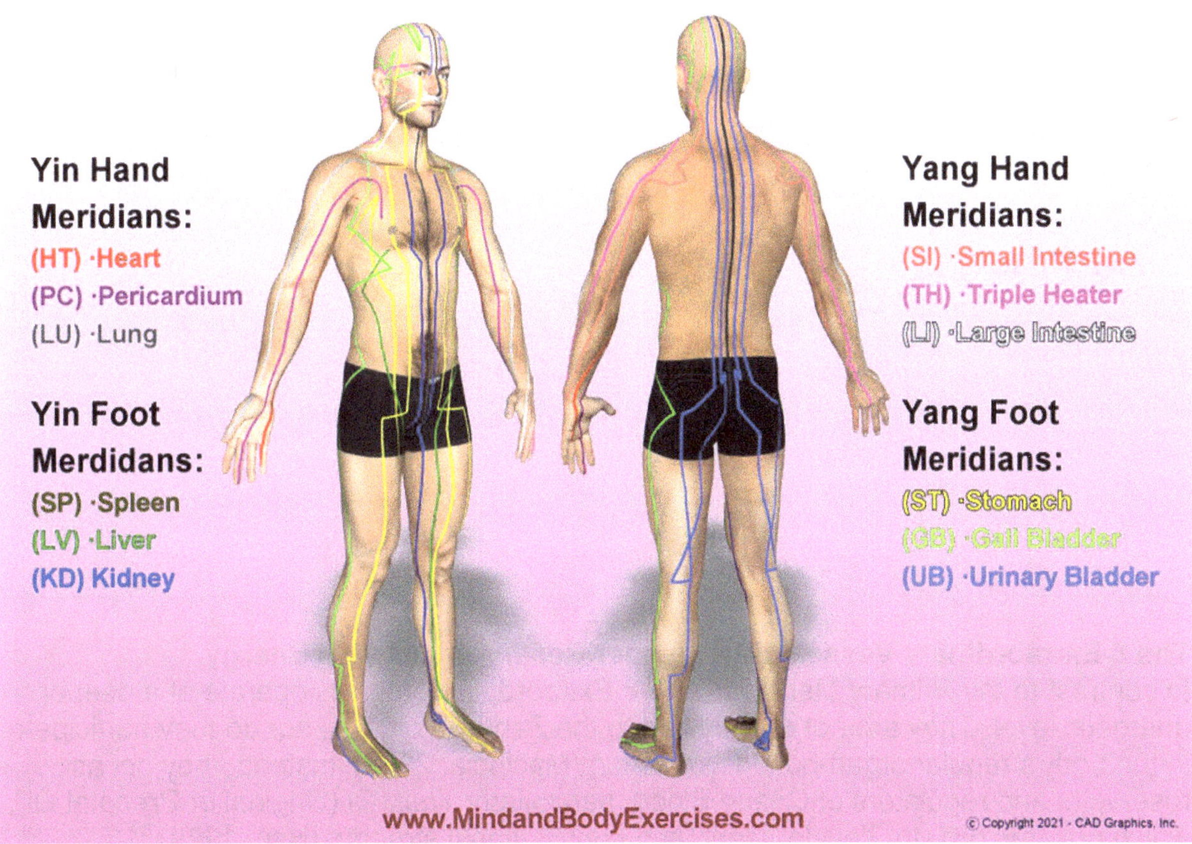

The 12 Primary Meridians: The Body's Main Rivers of Life

The 12 Primary Meridians are the foundational pathways through which ***Qi*** (vital energy) and blood flow to nourish the entire body (Deadman et al., 2007). These channels are intimately linked to the *Zang-Fu* organs of the five Yin organs (Lung, Heart, Spleen, Liver, Kidney) and six *Yang* organs (Large Intestine, Small Intestine, Stomach, Gallbladder, Urinary Bladder, and San Jiao/Triple Burner) (Maciocia, 2005).

Each meridian runs a defined, bilateral path along the body, connecting exterior regions (skin, muscles) with interior organs. This ensures that nutritive Qi (*Ying Qi*) and protective Qi (*Wei Qi*) are continuously circulated, supporting physiological functions such as immunity, metabolism, digestion, and mental clarity (Kaptchuk, 2000).

Because they regulate the daily functional balance of the body, the Primary Meridians are often the primary focus in acupuncture treatments and other therapeutic practices like acupressure and *Tuina* massage (Deadman et al., 2007). When these channels are blocked or imbalanced, symptoms such as pain, fatigue, or organ dysfunction can arise.

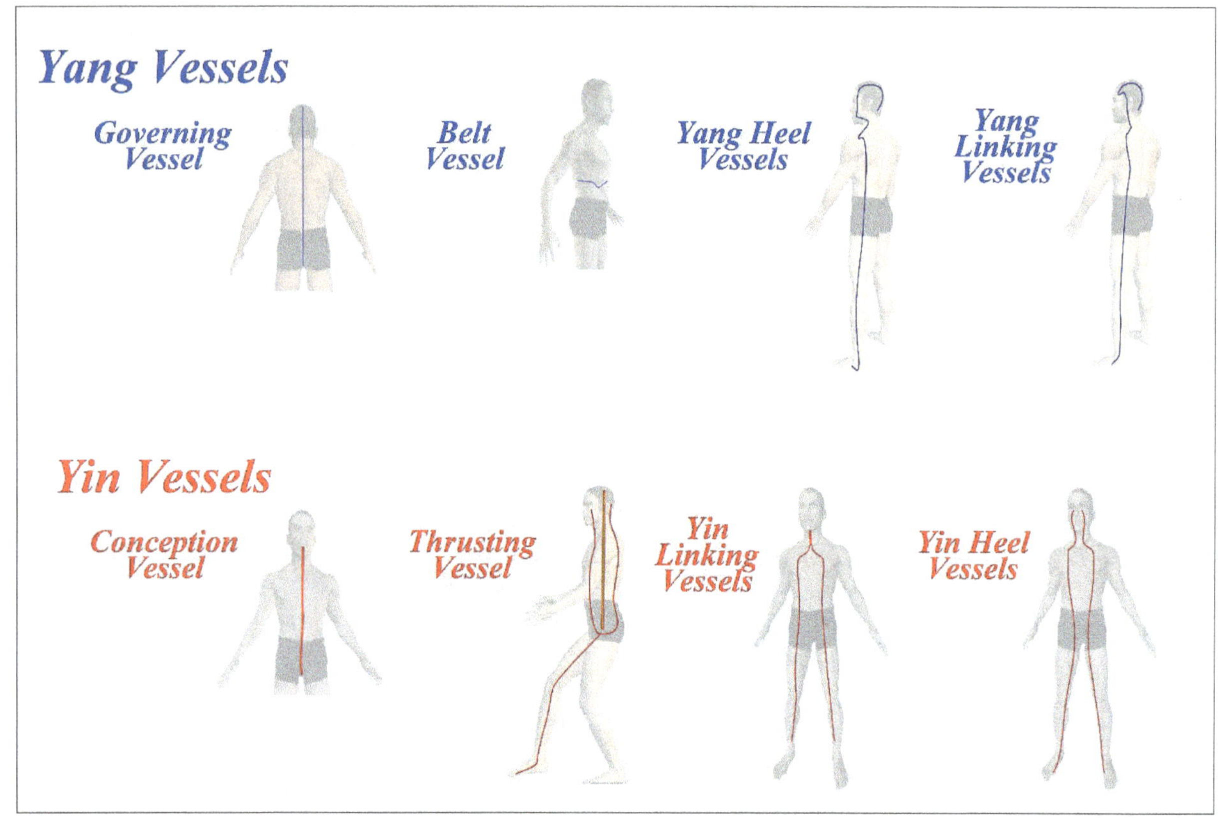

The 8 Extraordinary Vessels: The Deeper Reservoirs of Vital Energy
In contrast to the Primary Meridians, the 8 Extraordinary Vessels operate at a deeper energetic level. They are not directly tied to the Zang-Fu organs, nor do they participate in the body's regular organ-based circulation (Maciocia, 2005). Instead, they act as reservoirs and regulators of Qi and Blood, particularly *Yuan Qi* (Original or Prenatal Qi), which governs growth, development, and constitutional strength (Hsu, 1999).

While the Primary Meridians are paired and bilateral, several Extraordinary Vessels run along the midline of the body (such as the *Du Mai* or Governing Vessel and the *Ren Mai* or Conception Vessel), forming the body's central energetic axis. Others, such as the *Chong Mai* (Penetrating Vessel) and *Dai Mai* (Belt Vessel), regulate more specialized functions like reproductive health and structural integration (Deadman et al., 2007). The Extraordinary Vessels become especially important during times of:

- **Life transitions** (puberty, pregnancy, menopause)
- **Chronic illness**
- **Emotional trauma**
- **Deep constitutional imbalance** (Birch & Felt, 1999)

In such cases, they provide a reservoir of Qi and Blood that can be mobilized to restore balance and support healing. Advanced acupuncture treatments often target these vessels to address long-standing patterns of disease or to promote profound transformation (Birch & Felt, 1999).

Comparing the Two Systems: A Summary Table

Feature	12 Primary Meridians	8 Extraordinary Vessels
Number	12	8
Connection to Organs	Directly connected to major Zang-Fu organs	Not directly connected to Zang-Fu; deeper level
Flow of Qi	Circulates protective and nutritive Qi (Wei & Ying)	Regulates and stores Yuan Qi (Original Qi)
Pathway	Relatively superficial, follows defined body paths	Deep, more latent or reservoir-like pathways
Main Function	Maintains daily physiological function and organ balance	Acts as reservoirs of Qi and Blood; regulate overflow; integrate all meridians
Symmetry	Paired and bilateral (left and right sides)	Some are midline (single), others bilateral
Origin and Circulation	Continuous circulation in a closed loop	Originate from the Kidney/Yuan Qi level; flow in special patterns
Activation in Practice	Commonly used in acupuncture and daily therapies	Used in advanced, constitutional, or chronic condition treatments
Examples	Lung, Heart, Kidney, Spleen, Stomach meridians, etc.	Du Mai, Ren Mai, Chong Mai, Dai Mai, and others

The Dynamic Dance of Qi: Rivers and Reservoirs

One way to visualize this relationship is to think of the 12 Primary Meridians as the body's main rivers of energy flow (Kaptchuk, 2000). They nourish the landscape (organs and tissues) with a steady stream of Qi and Blood. In contrast, the 8 Extraordinary Vessels serve as reservoirs and aqueducts that hold, regulate, and distribute this energy as needed during times of surplus or deficiency (Hsu, 1999).

This layered system allows TCM to address health at multiple levels, from acute, surface-level imbalances to deep constitutional healing that shapes one's vitality, longevity, and adaptability (Birch & Felt, 1999).

Practical Implications for Wellness

For modern practitioners and wellness seekers, understanding this distinction helps guide personal practices:

- **Daily self-care** and lifestyle habits (nutrition, breathwork, basic movement practices) primarily support the flow of the 12 Primary Meridians.
- **Deeper practices** such as *Qi Gong, Nei Gong*, and meditative breathwork can engage the Extraordinary Vessels to cultivate life force and restore balance at a core level (Deadman et al., 2007).
- **Clinical interventions** (like specialized acupuncture protocols) can be designed to activate specific Extraordinary Vessels to address chronic or deeply rooted issues (Birch & Felt, 1999).

Conclusion

Both the 12 Primary Meridians and the 8 Extraordinary Vessels are essential components of the TCM energy system, working together to maintain health, resilience, and harmony throughout life (Maciocia, 2005). By appreciating their complementary roles, we gain a richer understanding of how traditional practices can support modern well-being in a profound and holistic way.

Opening & Filling of the 8 Vessels
(Taoist Yoga/Taoist Qigong
for internal and external strength training)
www.MindAndBodyExercises.com
1. Seven Stars Press the Earth
2. Divide Heaven and Earth
3. Standing in Ba to Push the 2 Poles
4. Twist Like a Rope
5. Crescent Moon
6. White Crane Points to the 7 Stars
7. Ride the Tiger
8. Natural Palm Points to Heaven
9. Embracing Moon at Chest" posture
© CAD Graphics, Inc 2018

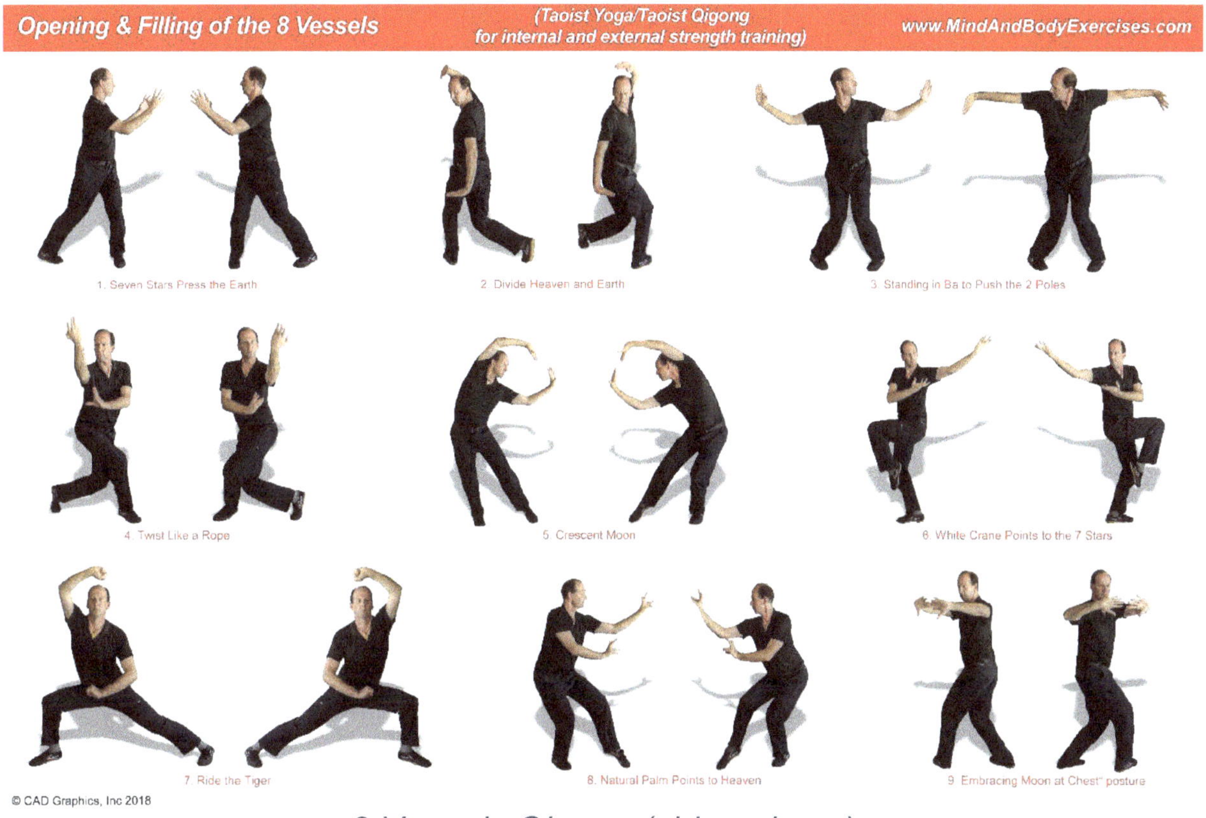

8 Vessels Qigong (ship pal gye)

References

Birch, S., & Felt, R. L. (1999). *Understanding acupuncture*. Churchill Livingstone.

Deadman, P., Al-Khafaji, M., & Baker, K. (2007). *A manual of acupuncture*. Journal of Chinese Medicine Publications.

Hsu, E. (1999). *The transmission of Chinese medicine*. https://doi.org/10.1017/cbo9780511612459

Kaptchuk, T. J. (2000). *The web that has no weaver: Understanding Chinese medicine* (2nd ed.). Contemporary Books.

Maciocia, G. (2005). *The foundations of Chinese medicine: A comprehensive text for acupuncturists and herbalists* (2nd ed.). Churchill Livingstone.

7. Spring has Sprung. Are You a Wood Element Constitution?

"Knowing others is intelligence;
Knowing yourself is true wisdom.
Mastering others is strength;
Mastering yourself is true power."
— Lao Tzu, Tao Te Ching

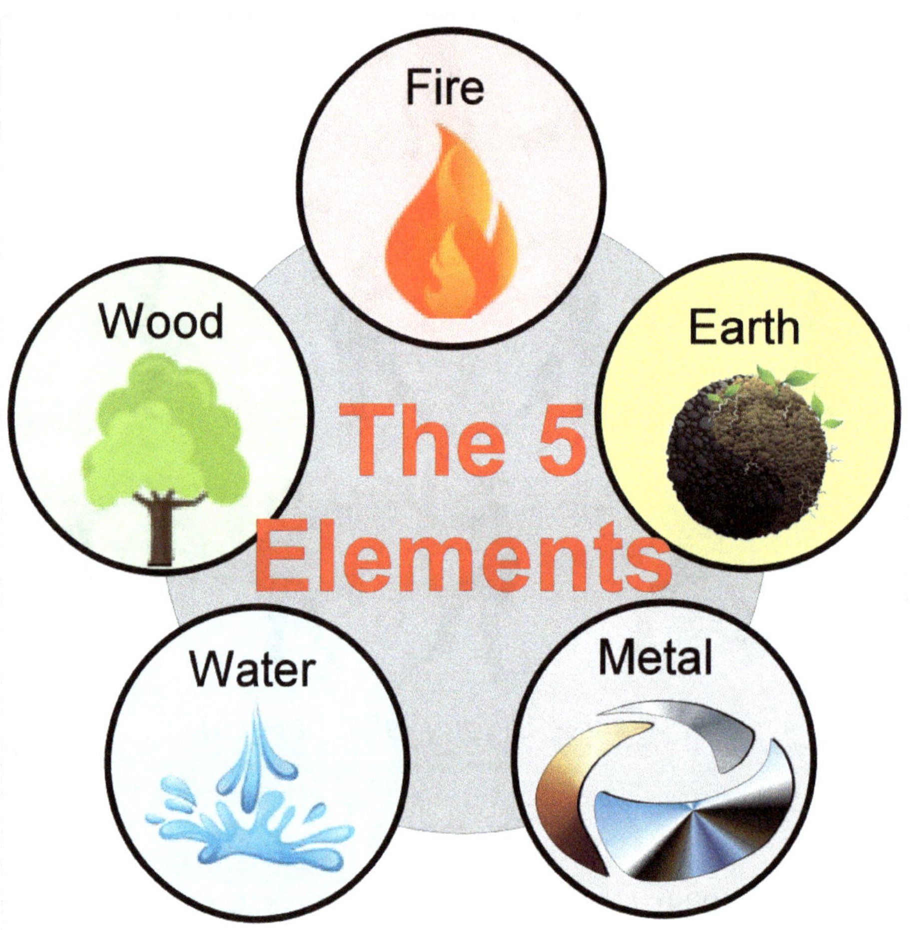

Knowing one's own constitution, as well as others in their life can help to better understand how and why people behave the way they do under certain situations. Some may see this concept as somewhat controversial or as a version of "profiling." However, this concept has been used for over thousands of years in various cultures across the world, such as with Traditional Chinese Medicine (the 5 Elements), Hippocratic & Greco-Roman Medicine (the Four Humors), Jungian Psychology, Tibetan Medicine (Sowa Rigpa), Western Biopsychological Models (Sheldon's Somatotypes). Ayurveda (Indian "study of life") and indigenous peoples across the globe.

The Wood Element in Traditional Chinese Medicine

In Traditional Chinese Medicine (TCM), the **Wood** Element is one of the five fundamental forces in the Five Element Theory, which explains the interconnection between natural phenomena and human life. Each element of Wood, Fire, Earth, Metal, and Water, corresponds to specific seasons of the year, organs, emotions, and physiological processes. Wood, in particular, is linked to the season of spring, the liver and gallbladder, shaping both physical and psychological characteristics in individuals with a "Wood constitution." The Wood Element is characterized by physical movement, ambition, and outward energy. While Wood types are dynamic and goal-driven, they must cultivate mental and physical flexibility and adequate rest to prevent stress and stagnation.

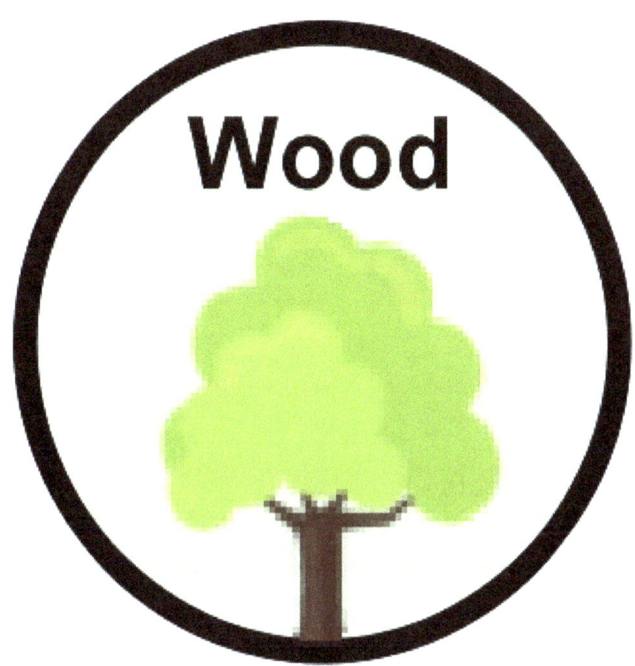

1. Physical Traits of a Wood Constitution

- **Body Structure:** Individuals influenced by the Wood Element typically have a sinewy, muscular build, often appearing strong and tall with an inherent sense of vitality.
- **Strength and Flexibility:** They usually possess endurance and adaptability, both physically and mentally, with a natural propensity toward movement and expansion.
- **Common Health Challenges:** Wood types may encounter liver and/or gallbladder-related concerns, including digestive disturbances, migraines, muscle and tendon stiffness, and detoxification difficulties. Liver Qi stagnation can also lead to menstrual irregularities or eye discomfort.

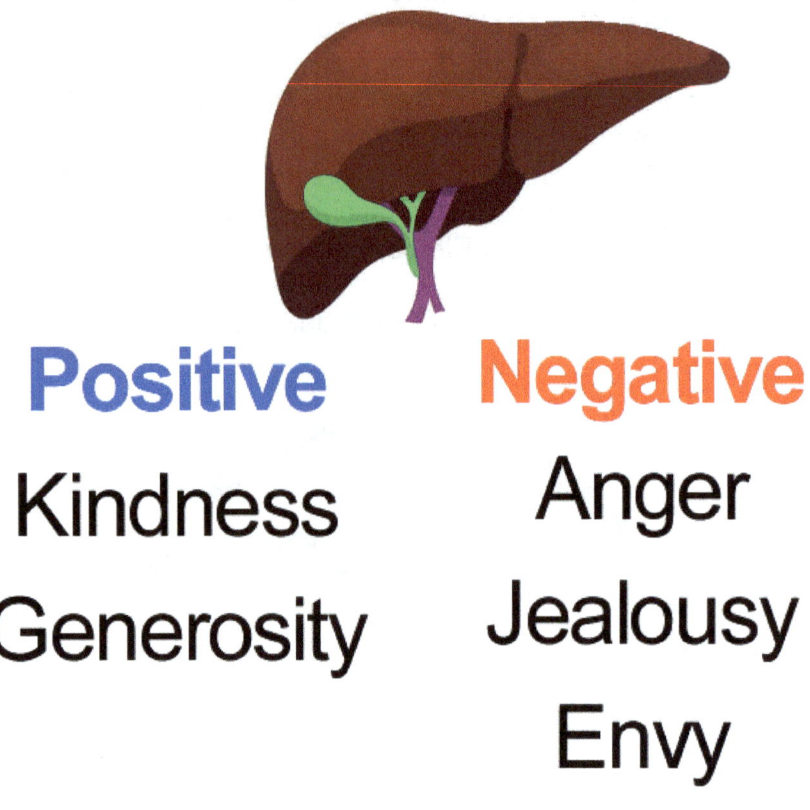

2. Mental and Emotional Aspects

- **Core Emotion:** The primary emotion linked to Wood is anger. When balanced, Wood individuals express healthy assertiveness, confidence, and determination. However, an imbalance can lead to frustration, irritability or struggles with managing emotions.
- **Personality and Leadership:** Wood types are often natural leaders, driven by vision, ambition, and a desire for growth. They excel in planning and organization, where they always seek progress.
- **Decision-Making:** They tend to be quite decisive and pioneering, eager to initiate change.
- **Emotional Imbalances:** When unbalanced, Wood individuals may become uptight, rigid, impatient, overly perfectionistic, and prone to burnout from excessive effort.

3. Spiritual Dimensions

- **Growth and Transformation:** The Wood Element embodies expansion, renewal, and personal evolution. Wood constitution individuals are often goal-oriented and deeply invested in self-improvement.

- **Purpose and Mission:** They often possess a deep connection to their life's purpose, inspired by justice, creativity, or a desire to bring new ideas into the world.
- **Bond with Nature:** Reflecting the qualities of trees and plants, Wood types of people often feel extremely connected to the natural world, drawing vitality and inspiration from outdoor environments.

4. Maintaining Balance in the Wood Element

To maintain harmony within the Wood Element, it is essential to cultivate their physical, emotional, and spiritual well-being:

- **Physical Care:** Regular body movement, stretching, and flexibility exercises help to support the liver and gallbladder. Regular consumption of liver-friendly foods like leafy greens also promotes internal balance.
- **Emotional Regulation:** Journaling, meditation, mindfulness, and relaxation techniques can help process emotions and reduce stress. Cultivating adaptability and releasing rigid perfectionism contributes to emotional equilibrium.
- **Spiritual Nourishment:** Making time to be present in nature, engaging in continuous learning, and setting personal growth goals can cultivate a sense of fulfillment and alignment.

Constitution	Characteristics
Fire	Extrovert, easily excited, center of party, the "kisser," difficult to calm down-exaggerates, sharp mental activity
Earth	Honest, kind, maternal, laid back, easily satisfied, aloof from the world, slow to respond to stimulus
Metal	Broadminded, wise, rule follower, aloof, righteous, confident
Water	Introvert, quiet observer, fearful, deep thinker, can be fear biter, consistent but slow
Wood	Extrovert, dominant, impatient, vigilant, enjoys moving/running, quick tempered, changes mind easily

8. Early Summer in Traditional Chinese Medicine

Fire Element, Circulation, and the Nervous System

As nature enters early summer, Traditional Chinese Medicine (TCM) views this vibrant season through the lens of the Fire element, a phase of maximum *Yang,* warmth, expansion, and communication. Fire governs not only the Heart and blood vessels, but also the nervous system, emotions, and spiritual awareness. This inner fire fuels both our physical vitality and our mental clarity. In this unique seasonal phase, the flow of *Qi*, Blood, and *Shen* (spirit), especially through the veins, arteries, and the Eight Extraordinary Meridians takes center stage.

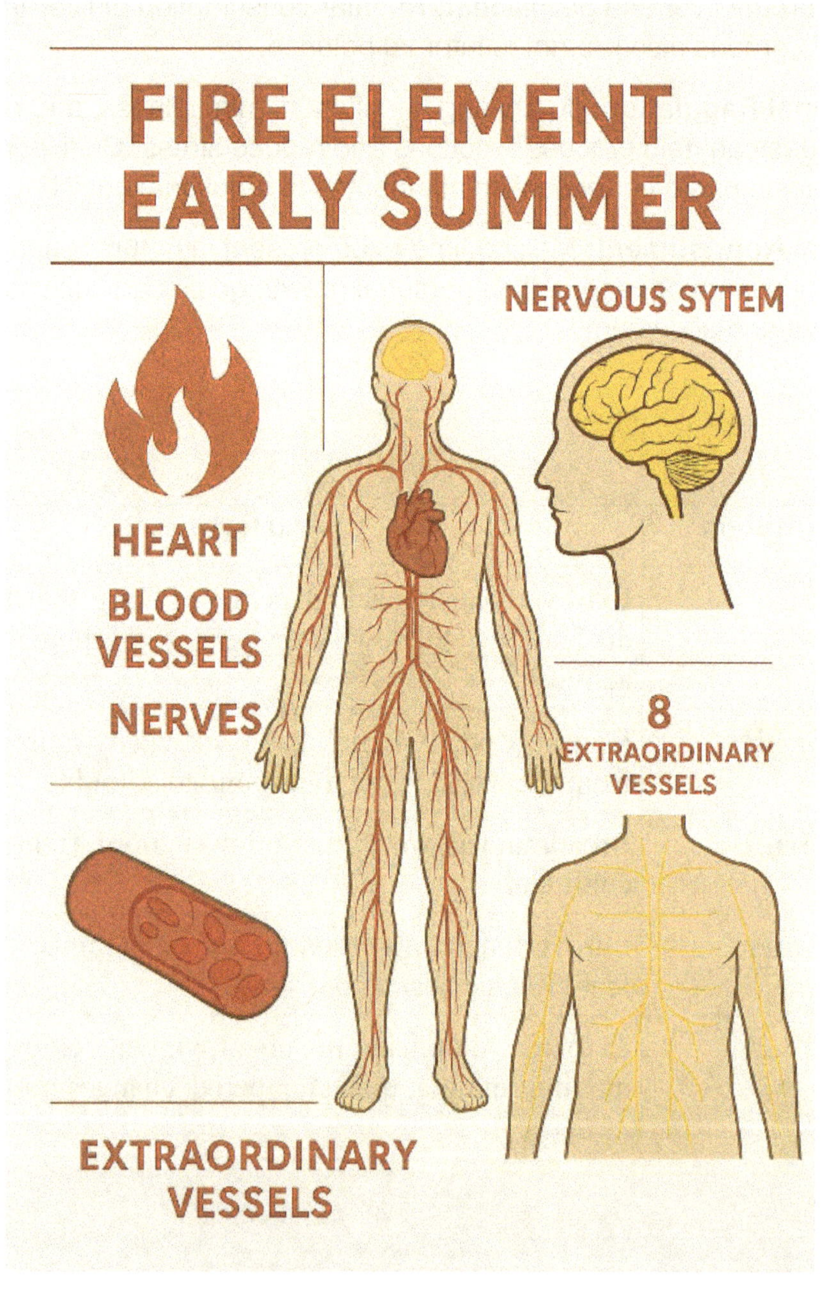

Understanding the dynamic between the Fire element, cardiovascular and neurological systems, and the deeper energetic channels allows us to harmonize body, mind, and spirit during this high-energy time of year.

🔥 Fire Element and Its Associations

In TCM's Five Phase (*Wu Xing*) framework, **Fire** is associated with:

- **Season**: Early Summer
- **Organs**: Heart (*Yin*) and Small Intestine (*Yang*)
- **Emotions**: Joy, enthusiasm, overexcitement, or mania
- **Body Tissue**: Blood vessels and the nervous system
- **Sense Organ**: Tongue
- **Color**: Red
- **Climate**: Heat
- **Direction**: South
- **Taste**: Bitter (Maciocia, 2005; Deadman et al., 2007)

Fire energy is expansive and expressive, symbolizing circulation, communication, and consciousness. When well-regulated, Fire fuels love, clarity, movement, and insight. When excessive, it can consume the mind and disturb the spirit.

❤️ Heart, Blood Vessels, and Nervous Regulation

The Heart (*Xin*) is considered the "Emperor" of the body, orchestrating the flow of Qi and Blood and serving as the seat of Shen (mind/spirit). TCM describes its functions as:

- Governing the blood and blood vessels
- Housing the Shen, which includes consciousness, thought, memory, and emotions
- Regulating mental activity and sleep (Maciocia, 2005)

The blood vessels, seen as pathways of both Blood and Qi, rely on the Heart's warmth and rhythm to remain supple and open. But TCM also suggests that nerve-like communication and coordination are part of the Heart's governance.

In modern integrative interpretations:

- The autonomic nervous system (ANS), particularly the parasympathetic "rest-and-digest" functions, mirrors the Heart's role in maintaining emotional and physical balance.
- Excess Fire may overstimulate the sympathetic nervous system, leading to agitation, insomnia, hypertension, palpitations, and anxiety.

- Deficient Heart Fire may lead to neurovegetative fatigue, poor concentration, and low vitality (Kaptchuk, 2000).

Thus, the vascular and neurological systems are harmonized through Fire's balance affecting everything from blood pressure to mood and mental performance.

🧠 Fire Element and the Nervous System

TCM may not anatomically label the nervous system as Western medicine does, but the concepts of *Shen, Yi* (intellect), and *Zhi* (willpower) reflect cognitive and neurological activity.

In early summer:

- Shen becomes more active and outward, seeking expression, connection, and joy.
- The *Du Mai* (Governing Vessel) linked with the brain and spine, rises in importance, guiding mental alertness and emotional regulation.
- The Fire element's influence supports neurotransmitter balance, sleep-wake cycles, and emotional processing.

From a modern neurobiological point of view, this aligns with the brain-heart connection:

- Heart Rate Variability (HRV), a marker of nervous system resilience, increases with parasympathetic tone, a goal of Heart-focused qigong and meditation
- Practices that balance Heart Fire can directly impact the vagus nerve, thereby stabilizing emotions and stress responses (Porges, 2011)

🩸 Extraordinary Meridians and Fire Circulation

The Eight Extraordinary Meridians function as deep energetic reservoirs, regulating circulation, constitutional energy, and emotional integration (Larre et al. (1996). In early summer, these vessels help modulate the Fire element's rise and distribute Qi and Blood in ways that nourish the whole system.

1. Chong Mai (Penetrating Vessel)

- Sea of Blood, linked to Heart and uterus
- Balances hormonal and emotional rhythms
- When Fire is excess: anxiety, chest oppression, uterine bleeding

2. Ren Mai (Conception Vessel)

- Nourishes Yin; anchors the Heart through calming fluids
- Connects deeply to Heart-Yin and Shen stabilization

3. Du Mai (Governing Vessel)

- Axis of Yang energy; influences brain, spine, and nervous system
- Becomes overactive when Fire flares upward, causing insomnia or hyperarousal

4. Dai Mai (Belt Vessel)

- Regulates Qi flow around the waist, harmonizes rising Fire from middle and lower burners

By supporting these vessels through breathwork, meditation, herbs, and seasonal living, we can help regulate the Fire element's effects on circulatory, emotional, and neurological functions.

🌿 Seasonal Strategies for Summer Balance

🔷 Qigong & Meditation

- Heart-centered qigong and the Inner Smile meditation bring Shen home to the Heart
- Breathing practices that lengthen the exhale can calm the nervous system and increase vagal tone
- Include "Cooling the Fire" meditations to harmonize Du Mai and Shen

🔷 Lifestyle Adjustments

- Avoid overstimulation, especially from social media, caffeine, or excess sun
- Go to bed earlier, maintain emotional equanimity
- Emphasize connection over excitement
- Prioritize joyful stillness rather than external thrill-seeking

🌀 Summary: Fire's Intelligence in the Body

Early summer is the season of Shen and circulation, a time when the Fire element stimulates outward movement, connection, and the full flowering of human potential. Yet this power must be anchored. Overexertion, excess heat, and emotional overload can disrupt the Heart, destabilize the nervous system, and drain the blood vessels and extraordinary meridians.

Through awareness, breath, and regulation, we can cultivate a sovereign Heart, a resilient mind, and an inner flame that warms but never burns.

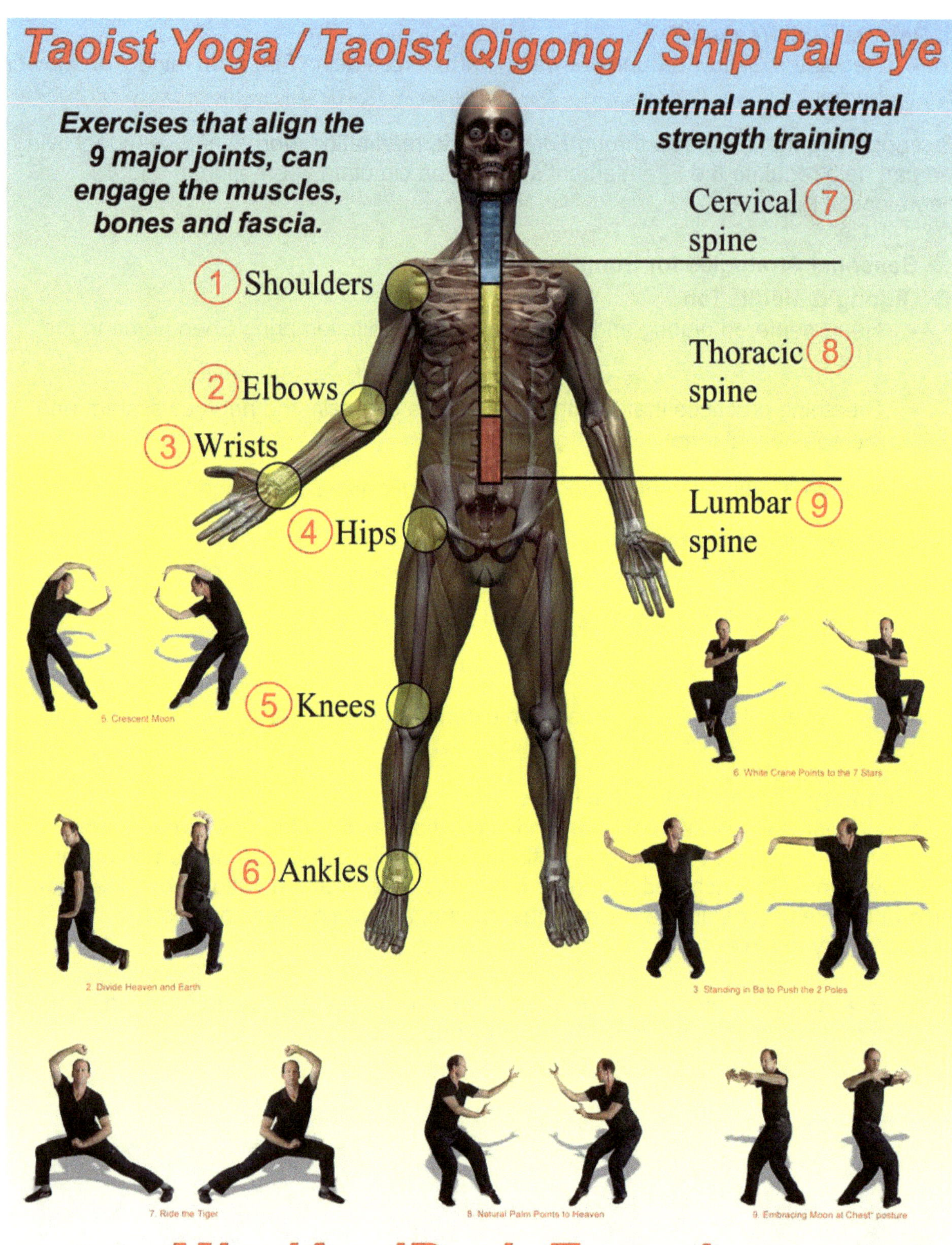
Taoist Yoga / Taoist Qigong / Ship Pal Gye
Exercises that align the 9 major joints, can engage the muscles, bones and fascia.
internal and external strength training
1 Shoulders
2 Elbows
3 Wrists
4 Hips
5 Knees
6 Ankles
Cervical 7 spine
Thoracic 8 spine
Lumbar 9 spine
5. Crescent Moon
6. White Crane Points to the 7 Stars
2. Divide Heaven and Earth
3. Standing in Ba to Push the 2 Poles
7. Ride the Tiger
8. Natural Palm Points to Heaven
9. Embracing Moon at Chest" posture
www.MindAndBodyExercises.com

References

Deadman, P., Al-Khafaji, M., & Baker, K. (2007). *A Manual of Acupuncture*. Journal of Chinese Medicine Publications.

Kaptchuk, T. J. (2000). *The Web That Has No Weaver: Understanding Chinese Medicine* (2nd ed.). McGraw-Hill.

Larre, C., de la Vallée, E., & Rochat de la Vallée, E. (1996). *The Eight Extraordinary Meridians: Spirit of the Vessels*. Monkey Press.

Maciocia, G. (2005). *The Foundations of Chinese Medicine: A Comprehensive Text for Acupuncturists and Herbalists* (2nd ed.). Elsevier Churchill Livingstone.

Porges, S. W. (2011). *The polyvagal theory: Neurophysiological foundations of emotions, attachment, communication, and self-regulation*. W. W. Norton & Company.

Part III — Traditional Therapies

9. Cupping Therapy vs. Bruising

Understanding Practice, Physiology, and Misconceptions

In today's wellness landscape, cupping therapy has re-emerged as a widely used modality for relieving pain, improving circulation, and supporting holistic healing. Despite its growing popularity, many people unfamiliar with Traditional Chinese Medicine (TCM) often confuse the distinct circular marks left by cupping with bruises from injury. Though they appear similar, the mechanisms, meanings, and physiological effects are fundamentally different. This article provides a thorough understanding of cupping therapy, its roots in TCM, its interpretation through the lens of Western science, and how it compares to traumatic bruising, to clarify misconceptions and deepen appreciation for this ancient practice.

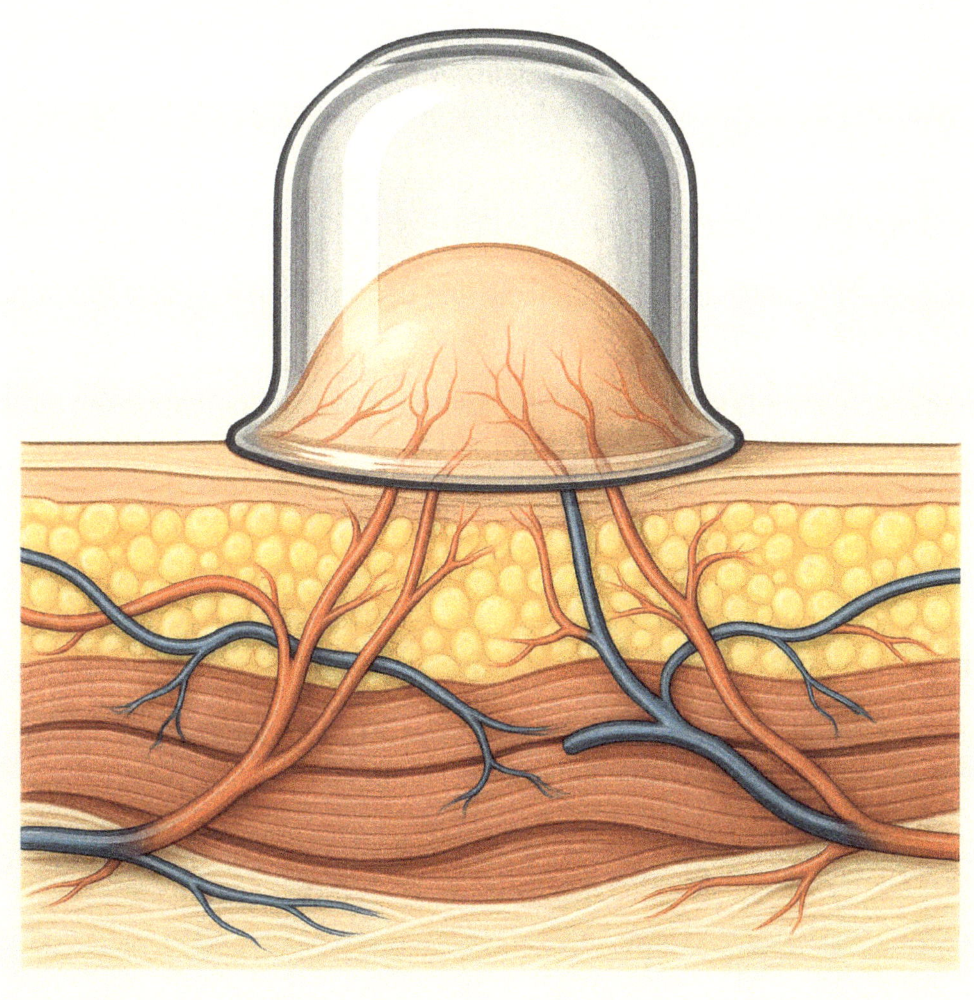

What Is Cupping Therapy?

Cupping is a technique that involves placing specially designed cups (glass, silicone, bamboo, or plastic) onto the skin to create suction. The suction pulls the skin and superficial tissue upward, promoting blood flow, stimulating lymphatic drainage, and mobilizing stagnation.

In Traditional Chinese Medicine (TCM), cupping is used to:

- Move stagnant qi and blood

- Expel pathogenic factors (wind, cold, damp)

- Open the meridians and facilitate energy flow

- Relieve pain, tightness, and toxicity

- Strengthen organ function by targeting specific meridian points

The Western Physiological View: How Cupping Works
Western medicine traditionally lacked a framework for cupping, but increasing interest has revealed several plausible mechanisms:

1. Increased Local Blood Flow – Suction draws blood to the surface, improving microcirculation (Lowe, 2017).

2. Fascial Decompression – Cupping lifts and separates skin, fascia, and underlying muscles, similar to myofascial release.

3. Neurovascular and Pain Modulation – Stimulation triggers responses through the Gate Control Theory of Pain (Teut et al., 2018).

4. Controlled Inflammatory Response – Mild trauma initiates a low-grade inflammatory response (Furhad et al., 2023).

5. Lymphatic Drainage – The pressure differential helps clear toxins and reduce swelling.

6. Parasympathetic Nervous System Activation – Can reduce stress and activate rest-and-digest mode (Harvard Health Publishing, 2016).

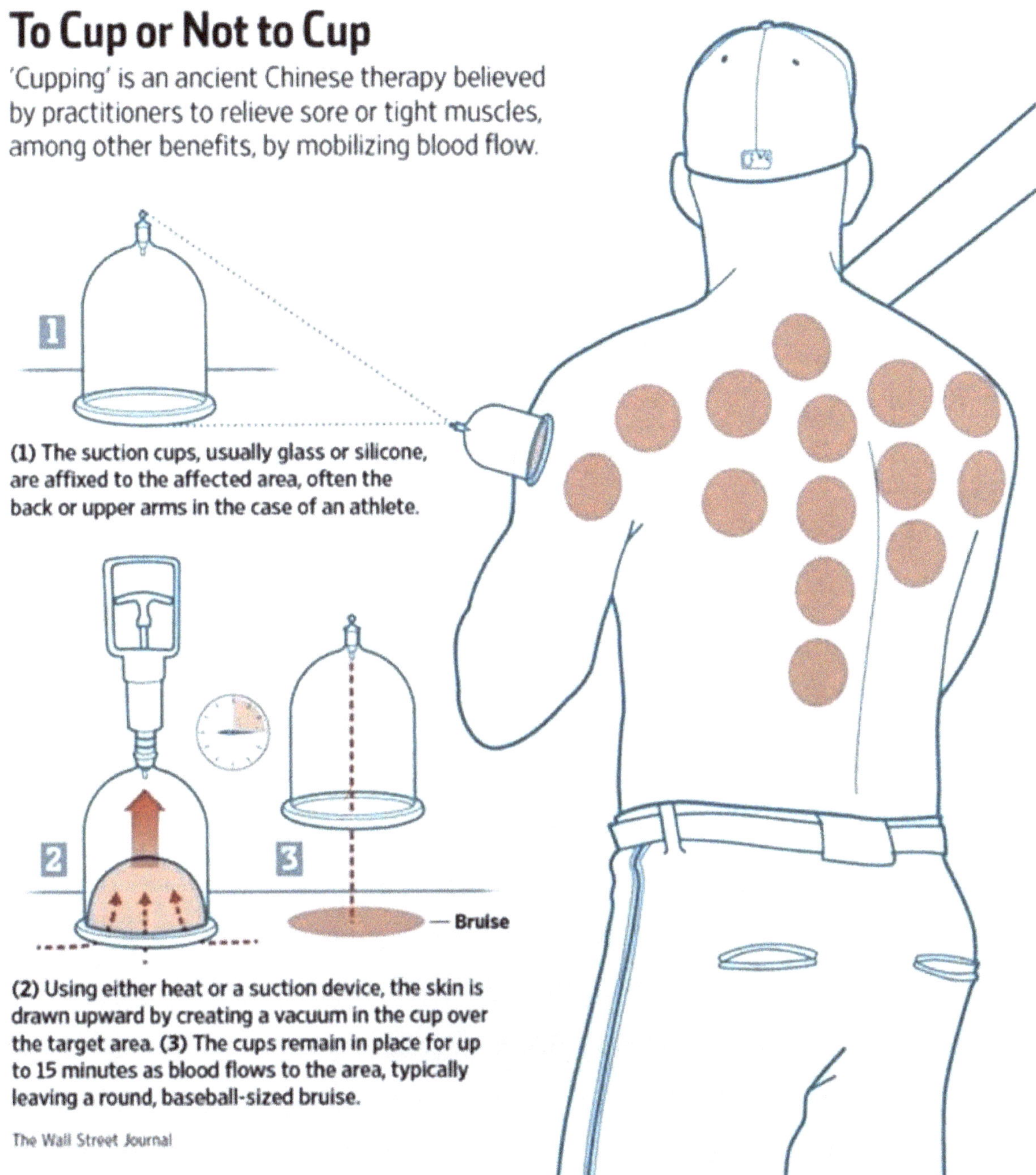

Types of Cupping

- Dry Cupping: Standard suction without bloodletting

- Wet Cupping (Hijama): Involves superficial pricking after suction

- Fire Cupping: Traditional method using heat to create vacuum inside the cup

- Gliding (Massage) Cupping: Cups are moved across oiled skin for deep tissue stimulation

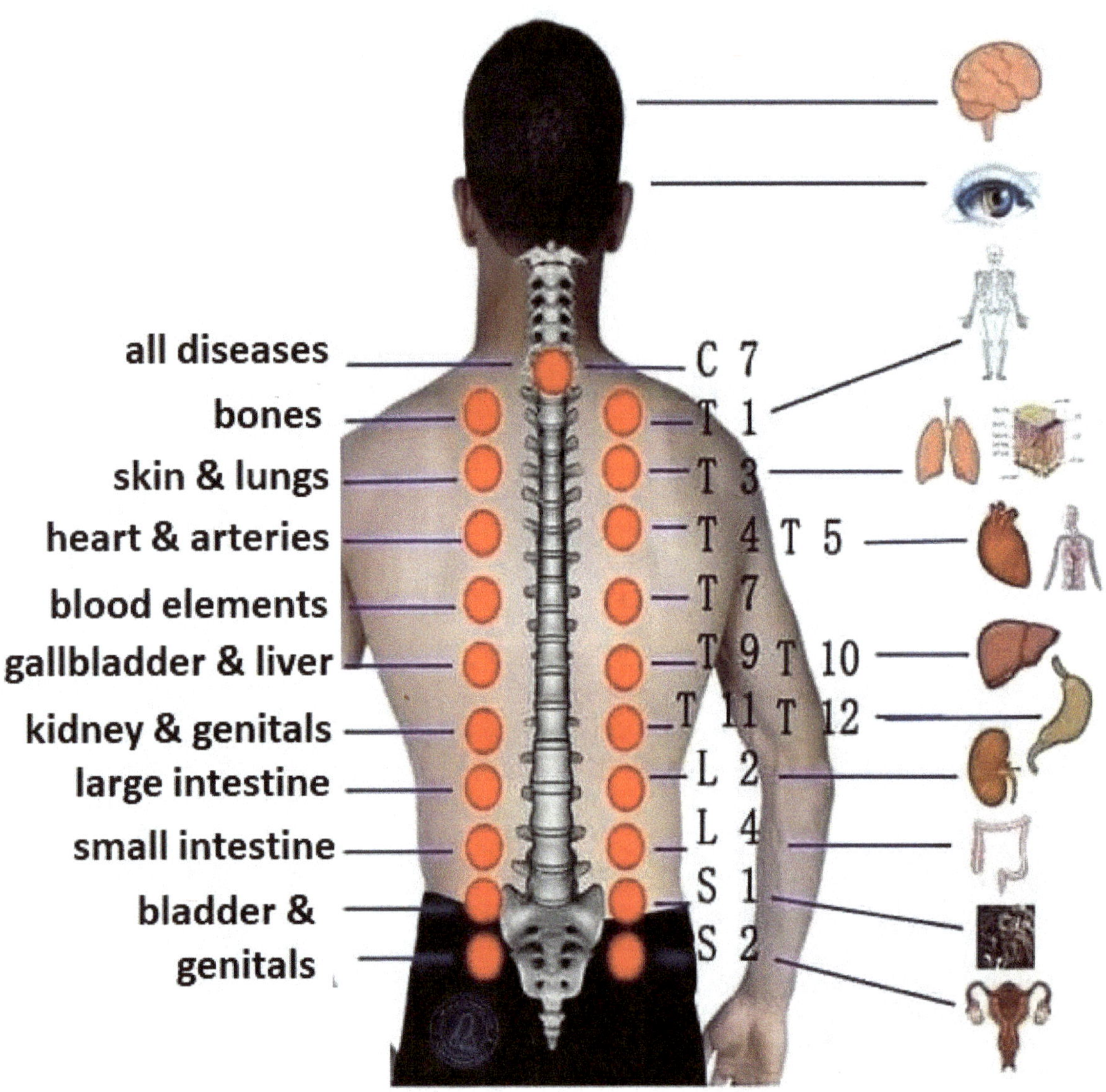

Understanding Bruising from Injury

A bruise (contusion) results from accidental trauma to soft tissue, leading to rupture of capillaries and pooling of blood under the skin. This causes pain, swelling, discoloration, and inflammation. Unlike the controlled effect of cupping, bruising often involves deeper tissue damage.

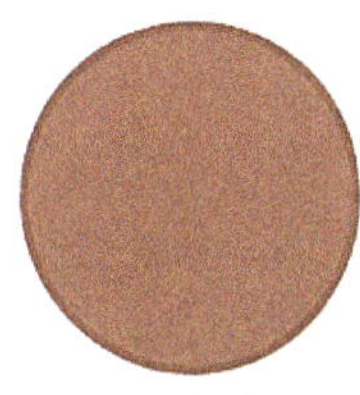	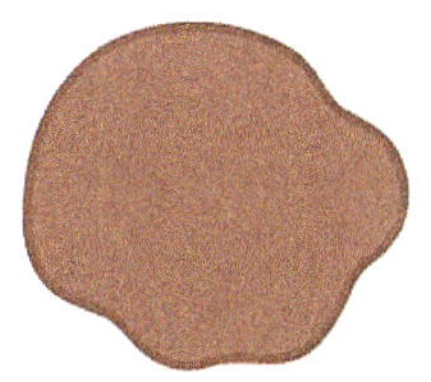
CUPPING MARKS	BRUISING (FROM INJURY)
Deliberate suction created by cups pulling skin upward. causing superfricial capillary ru-pture	Accidental trauma (e.g. bump, fall) causing damage to capillaries and leakage of blood under skin
Therapeute – To improve circulation, move stagnant qi and blood, release muscle ten-sion, and stimulate healing	No, result a previl of physical trauma or impact
Uniform, circular reddish-pur-ple marks; intensity varies ba-son stagnation level	Irregular in shape, colors change over time (red → purple → green/ yellow as it heals)
Usually minimal; some cliscom-fort may be telt during treatme-nt or afterward if tissues were tight	Often tender or painful, especially in the days immediately after injury
Duration within 3-10 days	May take 1–3 weeks to fully heal,

Comparison: Cupping Marks vs. Bruises
Cupping Marks vs. Bruises:

- Cause: Suction-induced capillary rupture vs. blunt trauma
- Intentional: Yes vs. No

- Purpose: Healing vs. Accidental

- Appearance: Uniform circles vs. irregular, color-changing marks

- Pain: Minimal vs. often painful

- Duration: 3–10 days vs. 1–3 weeks

Final Thoughts: Healing vs. Harm

Cupping is not a bruise in the conventional sense. It's a controlled, purposeful therapy used to stimulate the body's self-healing mechanisms. While cupping marks may resemble bruises visually, their nature, origin, and physiological impact are completely different. Understanding these differences demystifies this ancient therapy and makes it more approachable for those seeking holistic healing.

Side-by-Side Comparison: Cupping Marks vs. Bruises

Aspect	Cupping Marks	Bruises (Injury)
Cause	Suction-induced capillary rupture	Blunt trauma to tissues
Intentional?	Yes – therapeutic	No – accidental
Purpose	Detox, release stagnation, promote healing	None – consequence of trauma
Appearance	Uniform, circular, reddish-purple	Irregular, color changes over time
Pain Level	Minimal to none	Tender or painful, often with swelling
Color Pattern	Dark → fade gradually	Red → purple → green → yellow
Duration	3–10 days	1–3 weeks, depending on severity
Associated Symptoms	Relief, improved mobility, relaxation	Inflammation, soreness, potential joint restriction

References

Furhad, S., Sina, R. E., & Bokhari, A. A. (2023, October 30). *Cupping therapy.* StatPearls - NCBI Bookshelf. https://www.ncbi.nlm.nih.gov/books/NBK538253/

Harvard Health Publishing. (2016). What exactly is cupping? Harvard Health Blog. https://www.health.harvard.edu/blog/what-exactly-is-cupping-2016093010402

Johannes, L. (2012, November 12). Centuries-Old art of cupping may bring some pain relief. *WSJ.* https://www.wsj.com/articles/SB10001424127887324073504578114970824081566

Lowe, D. T. (2017). Cupping therapy: An analysis of the effects of suction on skin and the possible influence on human health. *Complementary Therapies in Clinical Practice, 29*, 162–168. https://doi.org/10.1016/j.ctcp.2017.09.008

Teut, M., Ullmann, A., Ortiz, M., Rotter, G., Binting, S., Cree, M., Lotz, F., Roll, S., & Brinkhaus, B. (2018). Pulsatile dry cupping in chronic low back pain – a randomized three-armed controlled clinical trial. *BMC Complementary and Alternative Medicine*, *18*(1). https://doi.org/10.1186/s12906-018-2187-8

10. Various Theories of Reflexology

Reflexology is based on similar principles to acupuncture as well as some types of massage. Our bodies are mapped by meridians of energy, or “chi” (pronounced “chee’). When we feel pain, discomfort or uneasiness, the flow of energy is blocked in some way. By putting pressure on parts of these meridians, the practitioner sends an impulse or signal all the way along it, which unblocks it and promotes the energy to flow freely again. There are various theories as to where the mapping of the hands, feet and ears corresponds to the different components of the human body. This post focuses mostly on hand positioning methods to achieve better health.

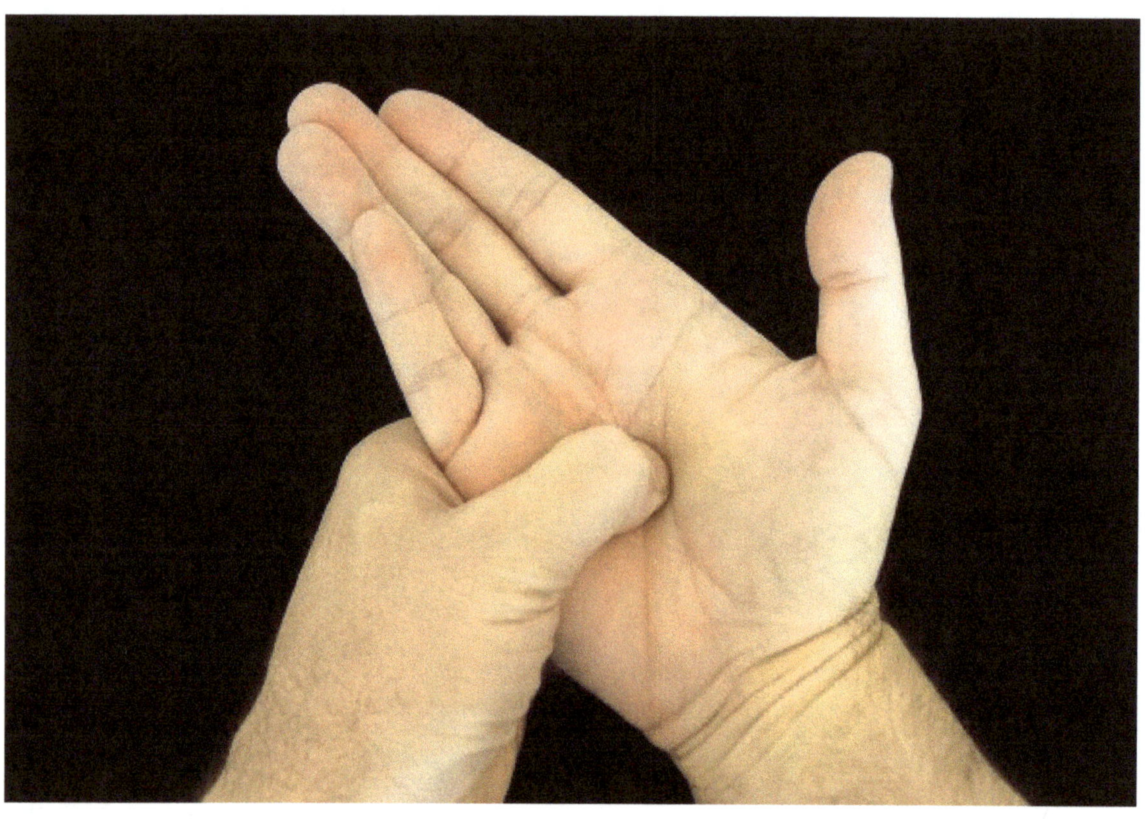

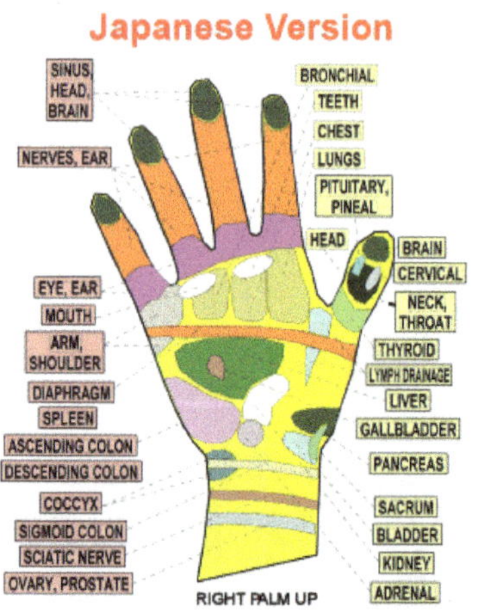

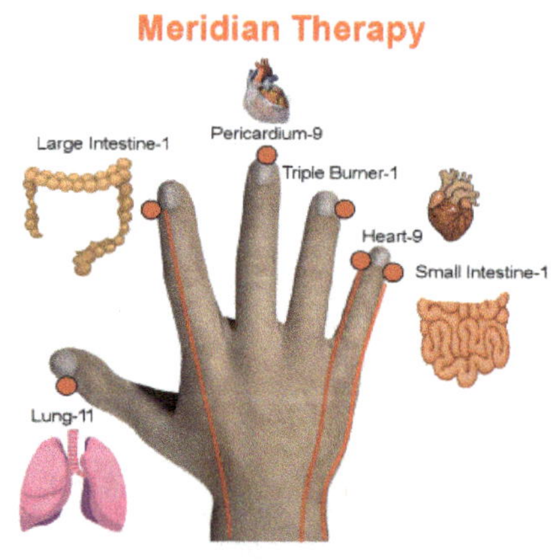

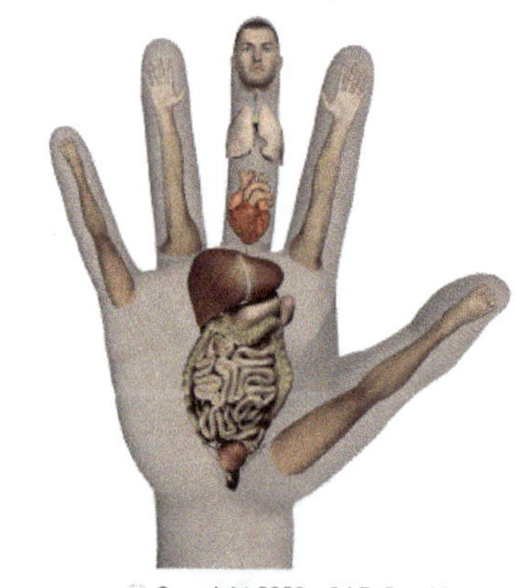

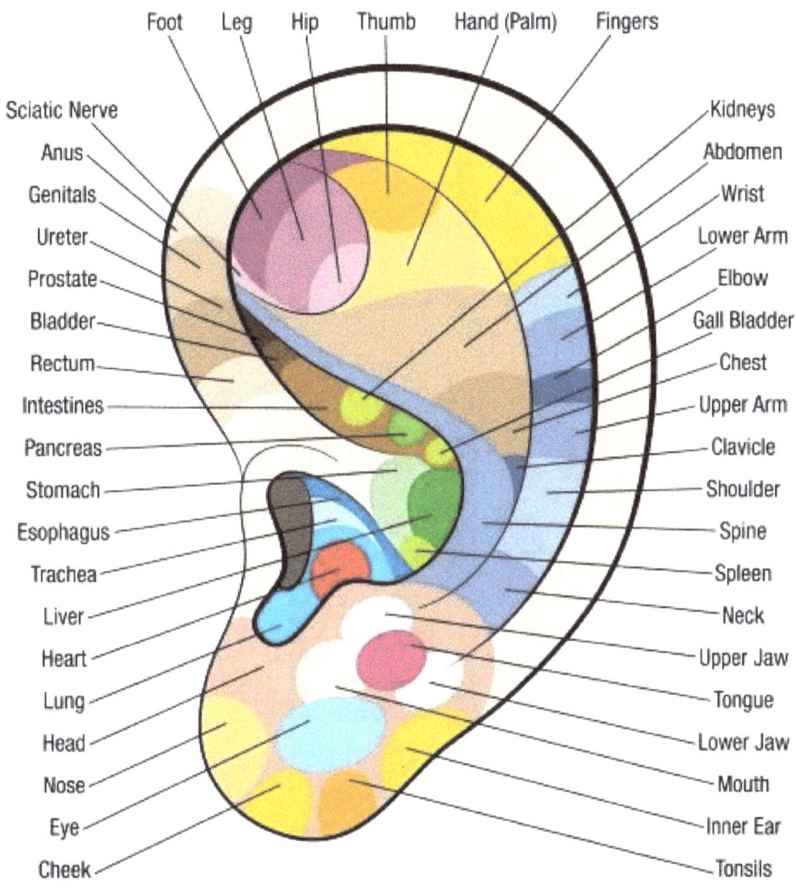

There are many types of reflexology:

- Reflexology of the feet, hands and ears (auricular therapy)

- Zone Therapy (5 zones corresponding to body components)

- Vertical Reflex Therapy (performed while standing)

- The Reflex Meridian Therapy (based on the 12 energy meridians)

- 5 Elements Reflexology (assessment & treatment based upon the theory of wood, fire, earth, metal & water)

- Geographic methods such as the Japanese, Chinese and Korean

Yin & Yang Acupressure Set

The Tourniquet Effect - These graphics illustrate the gentle twisting of the body and its various systems. The tourniquet effect restricts and then releases the blood and thus, energy flow to a specific organ, muscle or joint. Veins, arteries and organs are cleaned out, flushed with new blood and oxygen. The same events affect the joints, by flushing through and breaking down scar tissue while improving the quality of synovial fluids. This can help prevent and eliminate tendinitis and/or arthritis. These exercises should be executed in a relaxed and tranquil method. Relax the facial muscles and blur the vision. Most exercises should be done for 10 repetitions or more, before going on to the next in this series. Practice the massage of the both hands and wrist for 4-5 minutes before and after practicing the physical exercises.

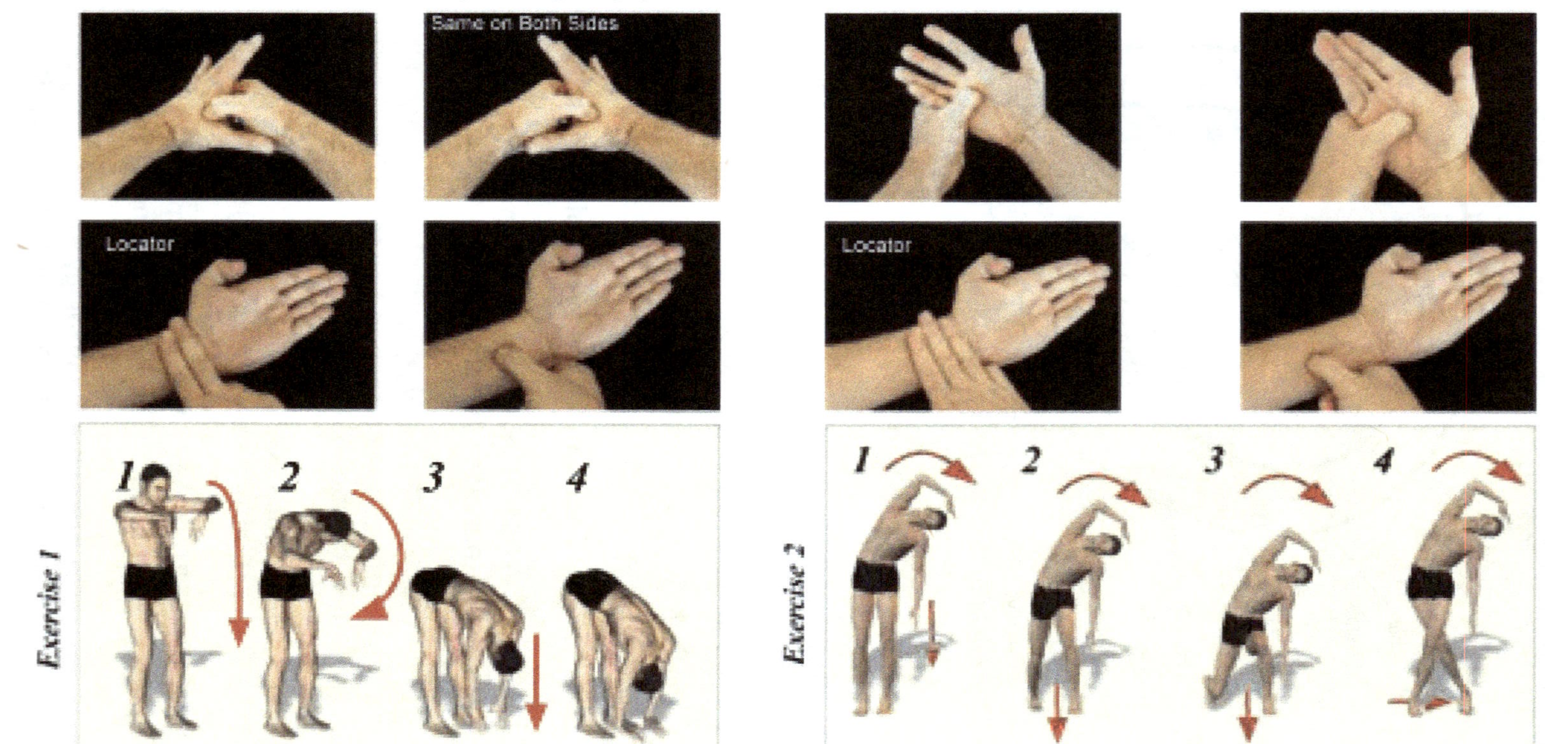

NOTES: **1-** hands hang loosely in front of face. **2-** chin to the chest as bending one vertebrae at a time while **3-** bending downward. **4-** Reverse by raising from the lower back, one vertebrae at a time.

Lower body variations: **1-** legs straight. **2-** leg back (bo stance). **3-** leg back (lunge position). **4-** leg behind (twisted stance)

11. Restoring Hand Vitality – Jing Well Acupressure

My Traditional Approach to Acupressure, Massage, and Herbal Therapy
As both a long-time practitioner and teacher of holistic wellness, martial arts, and Traditional Chinese Medicine (TCM), I have found that the health of our hands is often underestimated. Our hands connect us to the world, allowing us to create, heal, and express, but they are also vulnerable to stiffness, poor circulation, and overuse injuries, especially in our modern, screen-driven culture.

In my lecture and video presentation, I shared a traditional system of hand conditioning that I have personally practiced and taught for many years. This unique approach integrates acupressure, therapeutic trauma, herbal therapy, breathing techniques, and mindful movement. All designed to restore vitality, enhance flexibility, and promote whole-body energy flow.

https://www.youtube.com/watch?v=Vsk7z69df8I&t=1059s

A Philosophy of Health, Not Hardness
In the martial arts world, hand conditioning is often associated with building hardened fists and thick calluses. I take a different view.

The method I teach is not about brute strength or desensitization. It is about stimulating circulation, promoting healing, and enhancing energy (*Qi*) flow throughout the entire body.

Using bean-filled bags (I recommend soybeans, mung beans, or chickpeas), we create *strategic trauma* or gentle, controlled impacts that trigger the body's natural healing response. This principle, rooted in ancient wisdom, leverages micro-trauma to increase blood flow, strengthen tissues, and support overall wellness (Zhou, 2009).

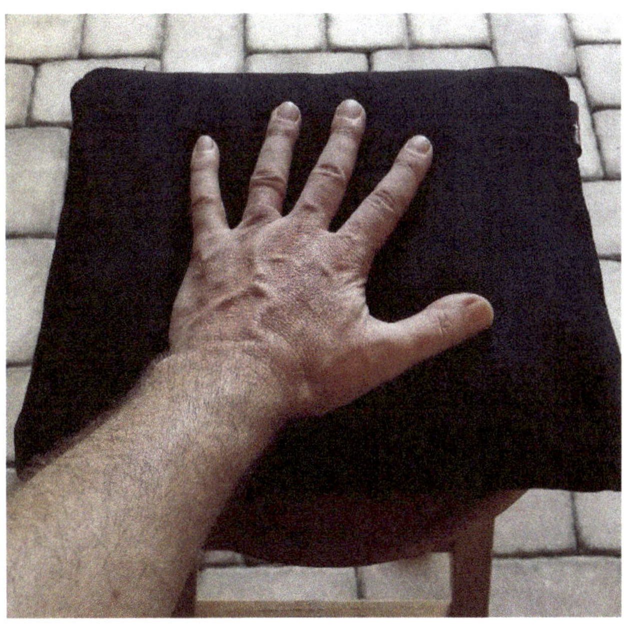

Hands as Microcosms of the Body

In my lineage or martial arts system, the hands are viewed as a map of the entire body, a concept validated by reflexology and TCM meridian theory.

- We focus on stimulating *Jing-well* points located on the fingertips—powerful gateways for regulating energy flow (Deadman & Al-Khafaji, 2007).
- I also reference Japanese and Korean reflexology maps, which beautifully illustrate how the fingers and palms correspond to internal organs and bodily systems (Ang et al., 2021).
- When we work the hands with mindful techniques, we influence not just the hands themselves, but the entire body and mind.

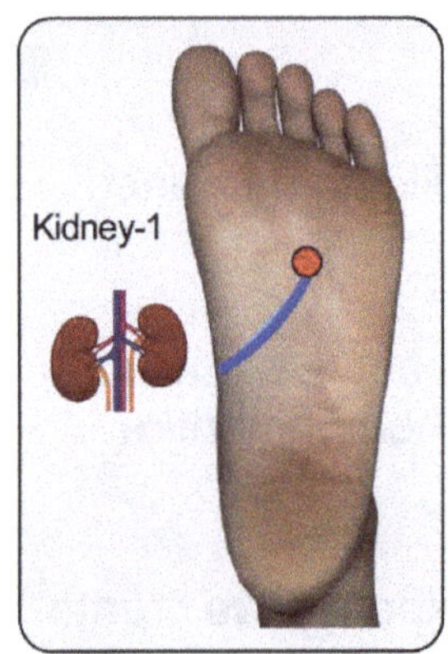

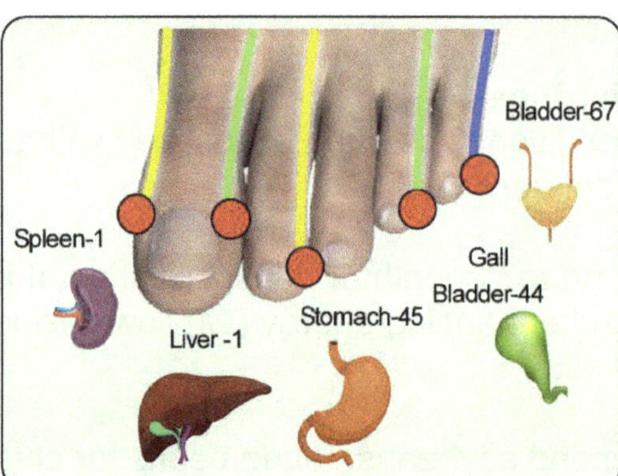

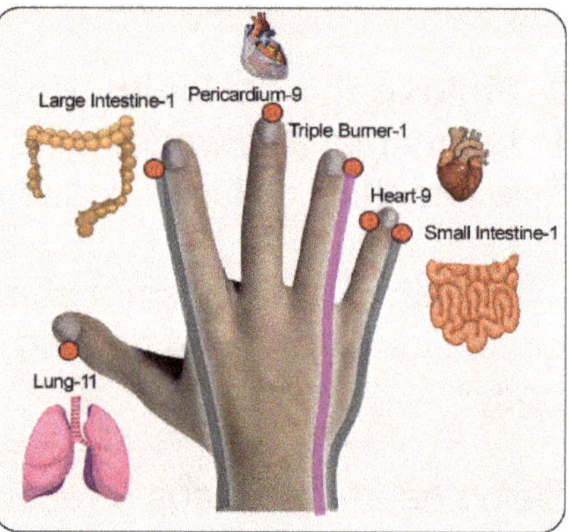

Breathing: The Missing Link

A key element in my lineage is Qigong (breath work), a deep, nasal breathing pattern combined with proper tongue positioning on the upper palate.

This breathing technique activates the parasympathetic nervous system, promoting relaxation, improving circulation, and harmonizing Qi flow (Sancier, 2001).

When combined with hand exercises, this breathwork turns a simple routine into a powerful integrative practice that nourishes body, mind, and spirit.

The Practice in Action

During my presentation, I guided participants through a progressive series of hand conditioning techniques, including:

- **Pinching, clapping, and crab-finger movements** to stimulate circulation and flexibility.
- **Percussion on bean bags** to activate Jing-well points and trigger micro-trauma healing.

- **Twisting, stretching, and massage** for the palms, knuckles, thumbs, and wrists.
- **External application of herbal tinctures**, which I personally formulate using apple cider vinegar, frankincense, and traditional Chinese herbs, to reduce inflammation and enhance post-exercise recovery (Xu et al., 2013). *(Note: these tinctures are for external use only and should not be ingested.)*

Real-World Applications
One of the most exciting aspects of this practice is its practical value:

- Certain finger acupressure points can be used to help revive a fainted person; a technique I demonstrate and encourage students to learn.
- Regular practice can reduce symptoms of arthritis, improve joint mobility, and enhance overall hand resilience, making it valuable not just for martial artists, but for anyone seeking greater hand health and functional longevity (Kim et al., 2015).

Balance Is Key
In my teaching, I stress the importance of balance and recovery:

- **Do not overdo the hitting exercises!** Allow at least one day of rest between sessions.
- Always follow with herbal application to soothe the tissues and prevent over-inflammation.
- Listen to your body. This is a lifelong practice, not a race for quick results.

This approach embodies the philosophy I teach in all of my wellness work: true progress comes from harmonizing stimulation with restoration.

Closing Thoughts
For me, this hand conditioning system is much more than an exercise routine. It is a gateway to whole-body vitality and a deeper connection with the subtle currents of energy that animate us.

By combining traditional acupressure, mindful breathwork, herbal therapy, and thoughtful movement, we can restore the natural vitality of the hands, which in turn enhances our overall health, energy balance, and functional well-being.

I encourage you to explore this practice with patience, mindfulness, and care. Your hands and your entire body will thank you.

References

Deadman, P., & Al-Khafaji, M. (2007). *A Manual of Acupuncture*. Eastland Press.

Ang, L., Song, E., Lee, H., & Lee, M. (2021). Acupressure for Managing Osteoarthritis: A Systematic Review and Meta-Analysis. *Applied Sciences*, *11*(10), 4457. https://doi.org/10.3390/app11104457

Sancier, K. M. (2001). Search for Medical Applications of Qigong with the Qigong Database™. *The Journal of Alternative and Complementary Medicine*, *7*(1), 93–95. https://doi.org/10.1089/107555301300004574

Starr, P. (2020). *Authentic Iron Palm: The Complete Training Manual*. Blue Snake Books.

Xu, Q., Bauer, R., Hendry, B. M., Fan, T., Zhao, Z., Duez, P., Simmonds, M. S., Witt, C. M., Lu, A., Robinson, N., Guo, D., & Hylands, P. J. (2013). The quest for modernisation of traditional Chinese medicine. *BMC Complementary and Alternative Medicine*, *13*(1). https://doi.org/10.1186/1472-6882-13-132

12. Reiki and its Acceptance in the US Healthcare System

American culture and society have greatly become more polarized on many issues. I see there is much more of a divide over the last 40 years between religions, spirituality, and secular practices. Reiki is a Japanese energy-based healing technique that uses an individual's energy force to help reduce stress, and anxiety and encourage relaxation not only for themselves but also for others. The method uses gentle touch and placement for healing and tries to improve balance in the body. Reiki has become more accepted and understood in some regions in recent years and consequently, more hospitals in the US. I found a few sources that indicated that Reiki is more accepted and offered in more progressive areas of the US, such as New England (Miles, 2019) the West Coast, and New York (McKnight, 2023). In other areas such as the Midwest, the Rust Belt, and the South, not so much. There are much more work and education that needs to transpire before Reiki will be truly accepted as mainstream by the US population.

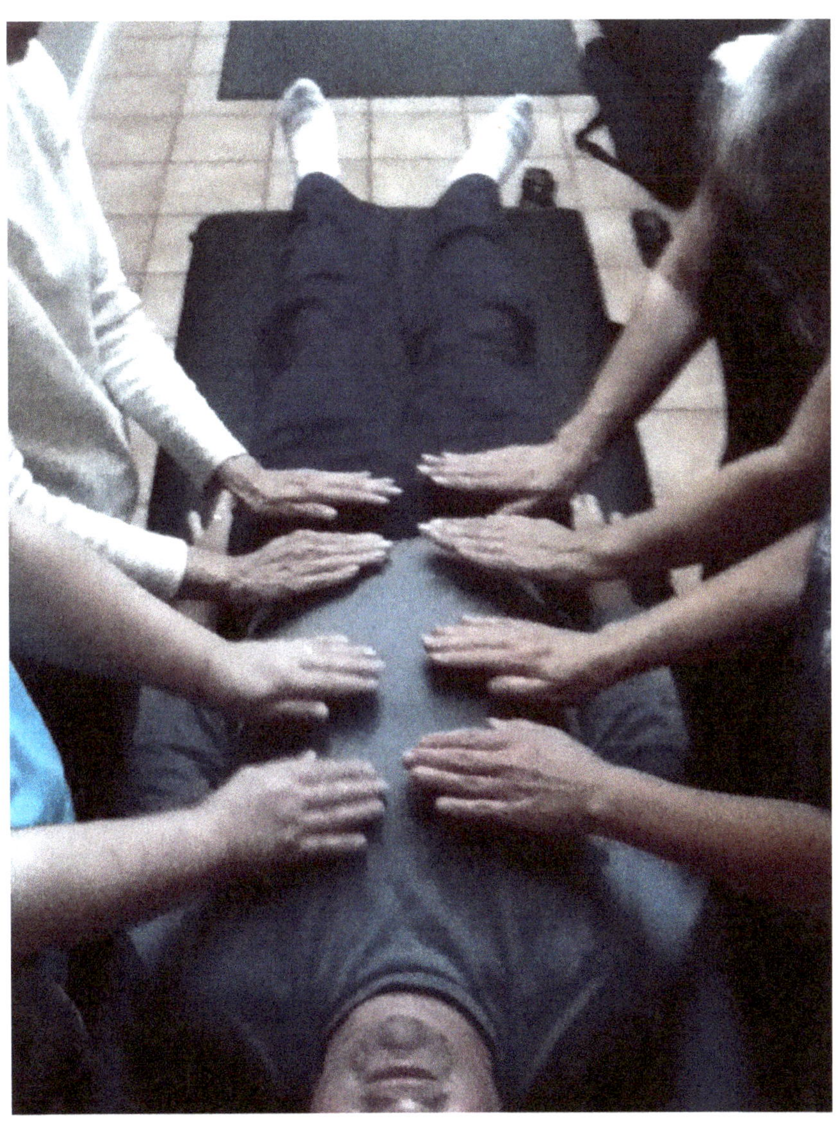

However, Reiki practice for some that are religious, may make sense and coincide with their belief in the power of prayer. For those who are spiritual, Reiki offers a non-religious option to connect to the divine or something greater than the self. For the secular, the basic premise of self-regulation through meditation and modulation of the nervous system (Miles, 2008) through managed breath control makes sense when applied to the Reiki concepts. With more studies, exposure, and education all three of these groups may embrace Reiki more in years to come.

I live in Orlando, Florida which has been typically labeled as being in the so-called "Bible-belt." This is a bit of an issue in that there are many people here, moving to or retiring here specifically to engage in the religious resources of many churches located throughout Florida. Not too much of a coincidence is that one of the largest healthcare providers in the US is Advent Health, which is a Seventh-day Adventist non-profit healthcare system headquarters in Central Florida. This particular religion does not support Eastern philosophy (Roman & Roman, 2022), making it extremely difficult to offer yoga, tai chi, qigong, Reiki, and other methods to its patients and the general public. I have tried hard over the last 30 years to work with their community outreach and senior wellness departments, where I have provided some lectures on bone health, balance, and stress management. I was instructed to keep my presentations on tai chi and qigong, within the guidelines of exercise and mindfulness breathing exercises. Administrators preferred for me not to get into spirituality, religion, or metaphysical concepts that may not coincide with the corporation's Christian mission, shared vision, or common values. When these healthcare providers do offer yoga or tai chi classes, they are usually just teaching physical exercises. From what I have found, Reiki is not offered much in Orlando except through private practitioners. This may change in years to come as I plan to become more involved in teaching holistic health seminars, for which Reiki will be a topic of my discussions.

Most people are aware that allopathic medicine is a very powerful and profit-driven model that generates about 4.1 trillion dollars per year in products, services, and employment (American Medical Association & American Medical Association, 2024). Anything that is free to learn/practice or empowers the individual to take control of their own health, is often labeled as pseudo-science or alternative, regardless of if other cultures have seen the benefits as legitimate, safe, and effective for thousands of years. "Safe and effective" often has a different meaning in the US where politics and profits often determine safety and efficacy. As the US continues to be more diverse in its assimilation of other cultures, we will continue to see more traditional healthcare practices come to be accepted in the US. Look how long it has taken for acupuncture, yoga, massage, Pilates, and other methods to achieve acceptance in the US. True knowledge lives on regardless of the day-to-day, year-to-year flippancy of a nation's viewpoints. If Reiki continues to offer benefits, studies will continue forward and hopefully eventually align with allopathic medicine, which would greatly broaden the acceptance within the general population.

One area of my concern with the potential for healing through Reiki practices is the potential karmic implications that may come about while attempting to help others. If someone is trying to heal by serving as a conduit to the Reiki energy, this is somewhat different than attempting to heal as a source of energy instead. It is my understanding from my own practices and study of Eastern cultures that often peoples' ailments, whether mental or physical, are manifestations of their own actions and circumstances. As a healer, one needs to be aware that many life lessons are meant to be learned, experienced, solved, and mastered firsthand. If not for the individual's own life lessons, but so as not to diminish the energy of other people. An example of this type of scenario is seen typically in the healthcare or first responder professions, where an individual may have good intent in helping another person, but that person often does not change their behavior or circumstances to avoid ailments or events, only to repeat them over and over again. The healer, helper, supporter, etc., often drains themselves physically, mentally, and spiritually while the patient, victim, or person in need becomes somewhat of an energy vampire consuming others' energy and good intentions.

References

Miles, P. (2019, September 16). Reiki in hospitals: An update by Pamela Miles, medical reiki master. *https://reikiinmedicine.org/*. https://reikiinmedicine.org/clinical-practice/reiki-in-hospitals-an-update/

McKnight, J. (2023, April 1). Full list of hospitals that use Reiki in the US. *Planet Meditate*. https://planetmeditate.com/full-list-hospitals-that-use-reiki-us/

Miles, (2008). (p.198) *Reiki, A Comprehensive Guide,* Penguin Publishing Group. Kindle Edition.

Roman, A., & Roman, A. (2022, February 24). *Yoga, Zumba, Les Mills, Te Fiti the Goddess of Creation, Disney Magic and the New 8 Laws of Health are all part of AdventHealth | Advent Messenger*. Advent Messenger. http://adventmessenger.org/yoga-zumba-les-mills-te-fiti-the-goddess-of-creation-disney-magic-and-the-new-8-laws-of-health-are-all-part-of-adventhealth/

American Medical Association & American Medical Association. (2024, April 25). Trends in health care spending. *American Medical Association*. https://www.ama-assn.org/about/research/trends-health-care-spending

Part IV — Breath and Internal Circulation

13. The Physiological Sigh and Daoist Breath Theory

Breathing is both an automatic physiological process and a foundational medium through which emotional regulation and somatic stability are maintained. Among the many respiratory patterns observed in humans, the **physiological sigh** represents a unique convergence of pulmonary mechanics, autonomic nervous system regulation, and traditional breath observations preserved in Daoist practices. Characterized by two sequential inhalations followed by a prolonged exhalation, the physiological sigh is an innate reflex that occurs spontaneously in healthy individuals and plays a critical role in maintaining lung function and nervous system balance (Del Negro et al., 2018; West, 2012).

While modern neuroscience and respiratory physiology have clarified the mechanisms underlying this breath pattern, Daoist and Traditional Chinese Medicine frameworks identified the functional importance of sighing centuries earlier, particularly in relation to Lung *Qi* regulation and emotional release. Examining the physiological sigh through both lenses reveals a rare alignment between classical somatic wisdom and contemporary scientific explanation.

Pulmonary Function and Alveolar Recruitment

From a biomedical perspective, the primary function of the physiological sigh is **alveolar recruitment**. During normal respiration, particularly under conditions of stress, fatigue, or restricted posture, small numbers of alveoli may partially collapse, reducing surface area available for gas exchange (West, 2012). Over time, this can lead to reduced lung compliance and diminished respiratory efficiency.

The physiological sigh counteracts this process through a brief second inhalation that increases transpulmonary pressure, allowing collapsed alveoli to reopen. This mechanism preserves lung elasticity and optimizes oxygen exchange, making the sigh an essential component of healthy respiratory maintenance rather than an incidental behavior (Del Negro et al., 2018).

Autonomic Nervous System Regulation

Beyond its mechanical function, the physiological sigh exerts a powerful influence on the **autonomic nervous system**. The prolonged exhalation phase enhances parasympathetic activity, primarily through vagal pathways, resulting in decreased heart rate, reduced sympathetic arousal, and rapid attenuation of stress responses (Porges, 2011).

Research in applied psychophysiology demonstrates that breathing patterns emphasizing extended exhalation improve heart rate variability and stabilize respiratory rhythm, contributing to reductions in perceived anxiety and respiratory discomfort (Lehrer et al., 2000). Because the sigh operates at the level of brainstem control rather than conscious effort, it remains effective even during states of emotional overwhelm or impaired cognitive processing.

Neurophysiological Basis of the Sigh Reflex
The physiological sigh is generated by respiratory rhythm centers located in the **medulla**, particularly the pre-Bötzinger complex and associated neural networks (Ramirez et al., 2013). These circuits integrate chemosensory feedback related to carbon dioxide levels and lung stretch, allowing the sigh to emerge automatically when respiratory efficiency declines.

This brainstem dominance explains why sighing is commonly observed during crying, emotional release, and moments of relief, as well as during sleep. It also explains why voluntary imitation of the physiological sigh can produce rapid calming effects when higher cognitive strategies are ineffective.

Daoist and Traditional Chinese Medicine Perspective
In Daoist breath theory and Traditional Chinese Medicine, sighing is closely associated with the **Lung system**, which governs respiration, rhythm, and the distribution of Qi (vital energy) throughout the body. The Lung is also linked to the ***Po***, or corporeal soul, which is sensitive to grief, shock, and emotional contraction. Classical medical texts describe sighing as a spontaneous mechanism through which constrained Lung Qi is released and chest tension is alleviated. The double inhalation observed in the physiological sigh can be interpreted within this framework as a restoration of ***Zong Qi***, the gathering Qi of the chest, while the extended exhalation facilitates the descent and regulation of Lung Qi. This process supports Lung and Kidney coordination, a foundational principle in Daoist internal cultivation and breath regulation practices.

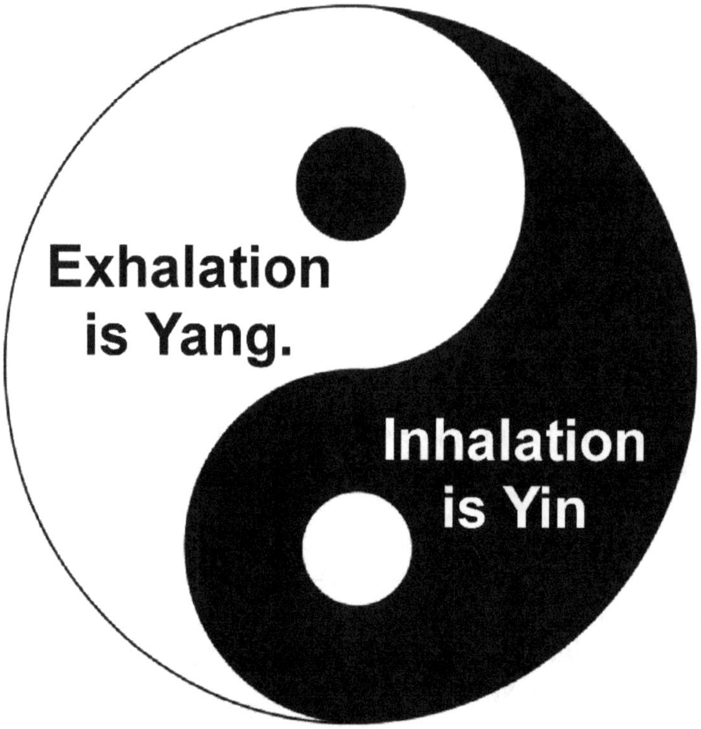

In Daoist breath theory, inhalation is Yin because it receives and gathers Qi, while exhalation is Yang because it releases and disperses Qi. Balance arises through their rhythmic alternation.

Dao Yin and *qigong* systems frequently incorporate a subtle secondary inhalation at the top of the breath, followed by a slow and complete exhalation. While historically described in energetic terms, modern physiology reveals that these practices align closely with alveolar recruitment and parasympathetic activation, suggesting that Daoist practitioners were observing functional outcomes long before their mechanisms could be scientifically articulated.

How to do a physiological sigh

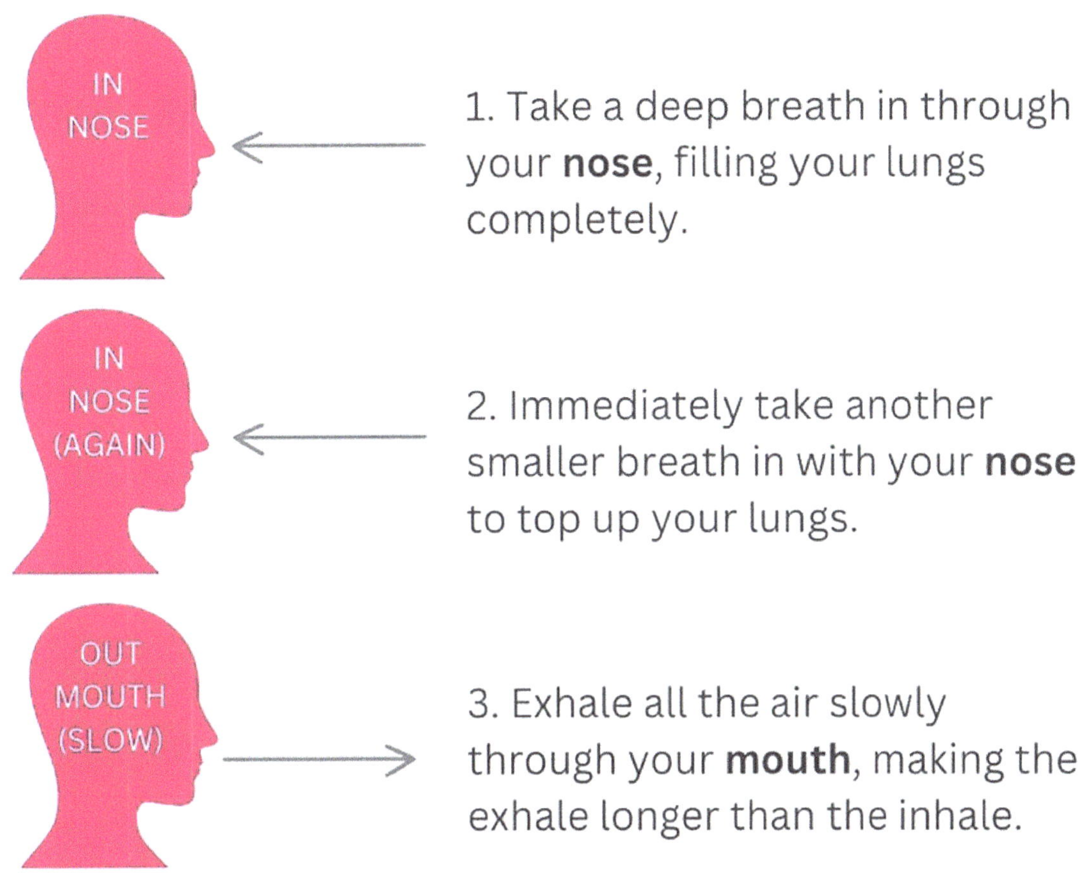

Integrative Application and Intentional Use

The physiological sigh can be intentionally reproduced as a practical tool for acute regulation:

1. A gentle nasal inhalation
2. A short secondary inhalation at the top of the breath
3. A slow, extended exhalation until comfortably empty

This sequence may be repeated one to three times and is best used as a reset rather than a continuous breathing pattern. Excessive repetition may lead to lightheadedness due to altered carbon dioxide levels.

From an integrative perspective, this method represents neither a purely mechanical intervention nor a symbolic ritual. Rather, it is a **functional reset** that simultaneously restores lung mechanics, autonomic balance, and somatic coherence.

The physiological sigh exemplifies a rare point of convergence between modern respiratory science and Daoist breath theory. Scientifically, it functions as an essential mechanism for maintaining lung compliance and autonomic regulation through innate brainstem circuits. Traditionally, it has been recognized as a natural means of releasing chest constraint, settling the Heart Mind, and restoring respiratory rhythm.

This convergence underscores an important principle in integrative health: some of the most effective regulatory mechanisms are not learned techniques, but inherent biological safeguards that can be consciously supported when needed. The physiological sigh stands as a compelling example of how ancient somatic observation and contemporary neuroscience can inform and enrich one another.

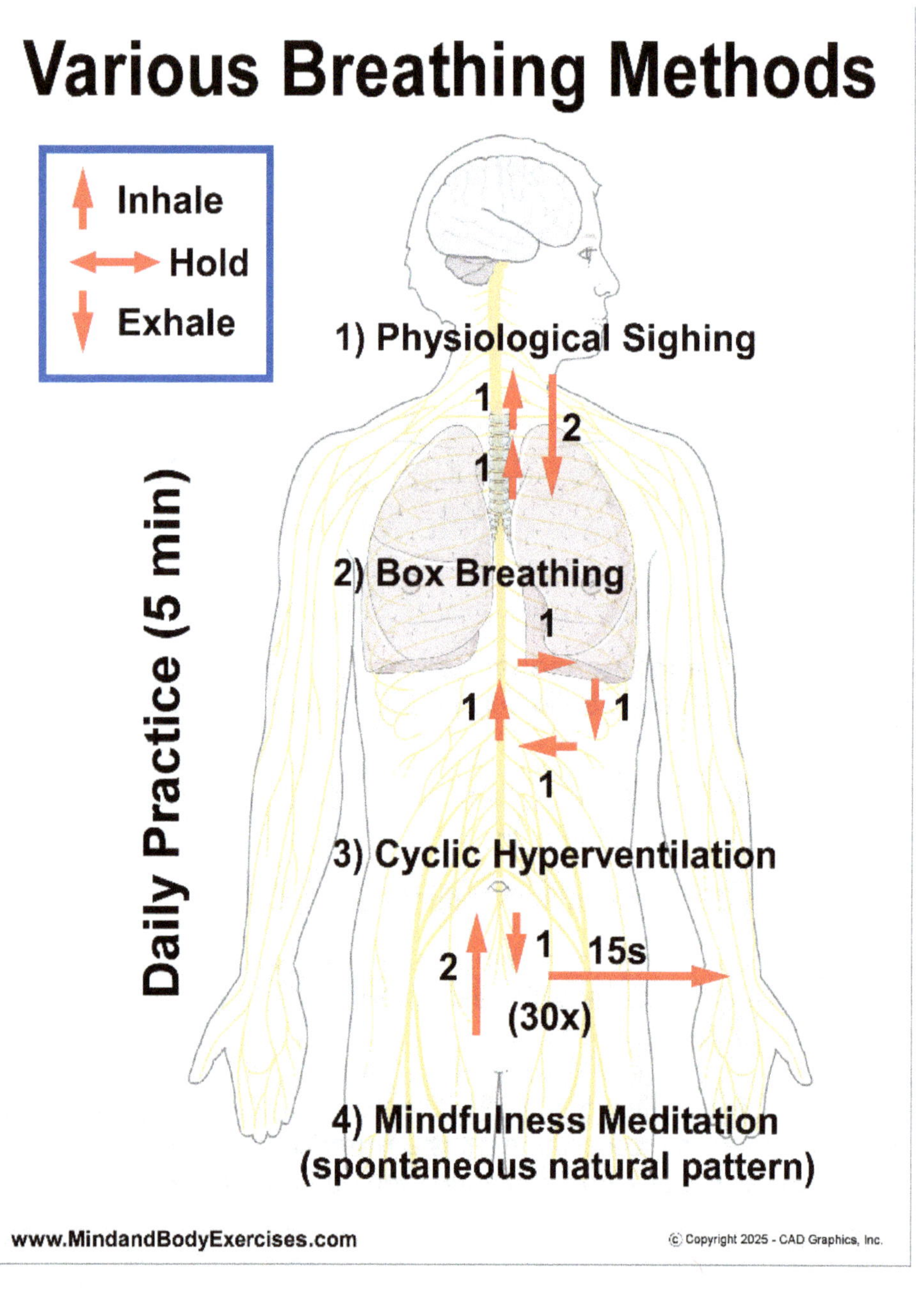

References

Balban, M. Y., Neri, E., Kogon, M. M., Weed, L., Nouriani, B., Jo, B., Holl, G., Zeitzer, J. M., Spiegel, D., & Huberman, A. D. (2023). Brief structured respiration practices enhance mood and reduce physiological arousal. *Cell Reports Medicine*, *4*(1), 100895. https://doi.org/10.1016/j.xcrm.2022.100895

Del Negro, C. A., Funk, G. D., & Feldman, J. L. (2018). Breathing matters. *Nature Reviews Neuroscience, 19*(6), 351–367. https://doi.org/10.1038/s41583-018-0003-6

Lehrer, P. M., Vaschillo, E., & Vaschillo, B. (2000). Resonant frequency biofeedback training to increase cardiac variability. *Applied Psychophysiology and Biofeedback, 25*(3), 177–191. https://doi.org/10.1023/A:1009554825745

Porges, S. W. (2011). *The polyvagal theory: Neurophysiological foundations of emotions, attachment, communication, and self-regulation*. W. W. Norton & Company.

Li, P., Janczewski, W. A., Yackle, K., Kam, K., Pagliardini, S., Krasnow, M. A., & Feldman, J. L. (2016). The peptidergic control circuit for sighing. *Nature, 530*(7590), 293–297. https://doi.org/10.1038/nature16964

West, J. B. (2012). *Respiratory physiology: The essentials* (9th ed.). Lippincott Williams & Wilkins.

14. Qigong – A Way to Heal the Mind, By Engaging the Body

This is a continuation of my previous post of how we can use knowledge within our thoughts to help to heal the ill, injured, damaged or traumatized human mind and body. Knowledge such as nutrition, appropriate exercise, management of sleep and healthy social relationships. This article delves deeper into the practice of Qigong or breath work, in order to help heal our body by using knowledge and conversely heal the mind by using physical exercises.

No need for a gym membership, a mat, special equipment or special clothing. Just some time, effort and a willingness to learn something different. Qigong practice is a solution to the current health care crisis, where we have seen a drastic increase in diabetes, obesity, depression, anxiety, stress, suicide and so many other mental and physically related health issues. Would it not be wise to at least consider preventing these ailments in the first place rather than using questionable pharmaceuticals and therapies after the fact? Folks, the horse has been out of the barn for many decades now. If government leaders, medical professionals, school boards and parents were to actually promote and encourage physical exercise, good nutrition, meditation and self-responsibility we might have a much different looking nation. Plant good seeds, no? Of course, there will be some that look at Eastern methods of healthcare such as yoga, tai chi, qigong and meditation as that "weird stuff" that they don't want their kids exposed to. So be it. Then maybe they can "do something" to fix all that ails our once great country.

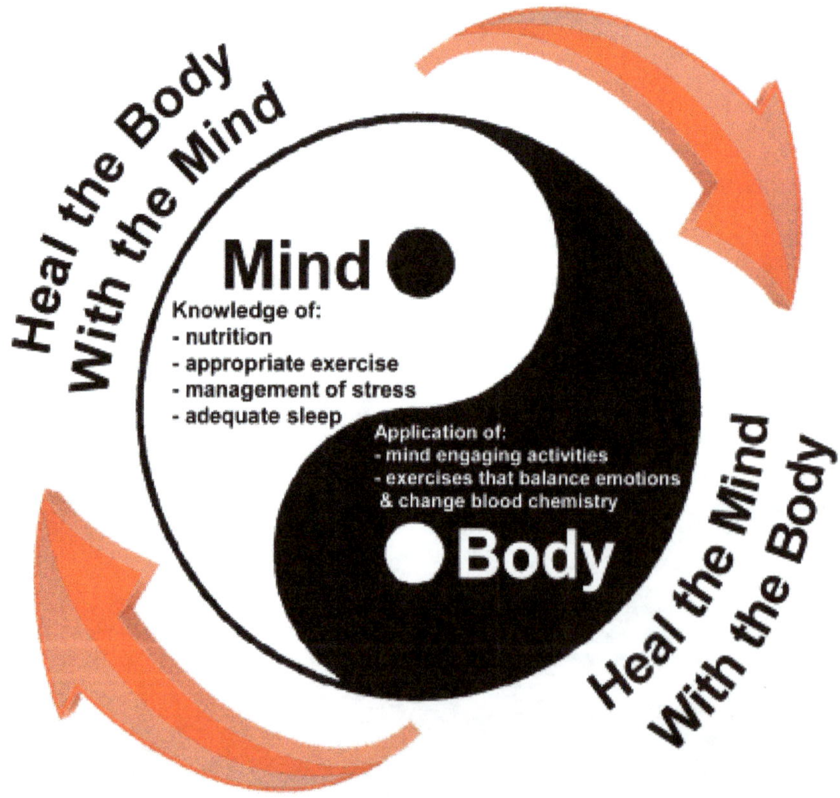

Qi pronounced "chee," means energy. You may see it spelled "Chi" or even "Ki" in Japanese, but they all carry the same meaning. Qi is the energy of the body, of the meridians, of food, of the universe. While it may seem a nebulous topic, there are refined theories regarding the different types of Qi within the body, the creation and actions of Qi, and consequently, ways to determine where imbalances may arise. "Gong" or "Kung" means work or diligent effort. So, qigong translates to "breath work." Qigong or Chi Kung is breathing exercises, with little or no body movement, can be practiced while sitting, standing or moving, Regulation of the breath can adjust the brain waves to the Alpha state. When the mind is relaxed, the body chemistry changes and promotes natural healing. With deliberate regulated breaths, one is able to relax the deep skeletal muscles working outward, while releasing tension accumulated within the muscles, organs and nerves. Whereas conventional physical exercise can deplete energy, Qigong helps to replenish your natural energy.

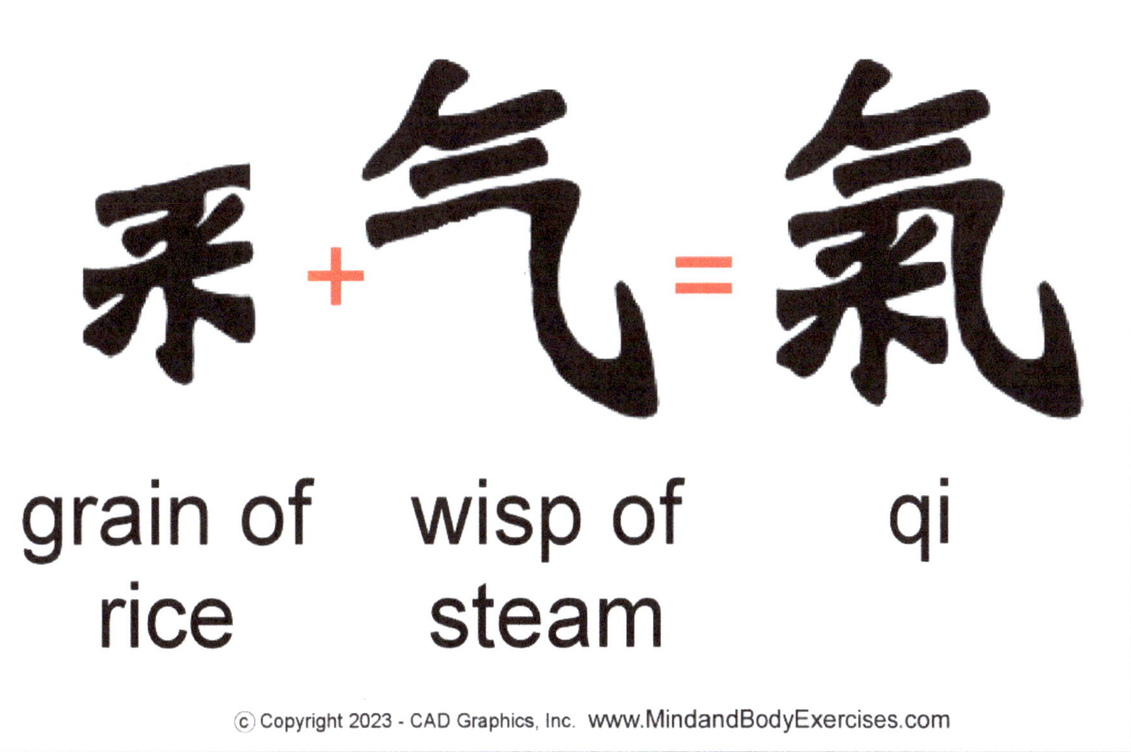

Qigong shares the same branch of origin as yoga. Both systems have sitting, standing and moving exercises with their respective curriculum. Both systems have a strong observance of the breathing mechanism and how it helps to balance out the mind, body and for some, spiritually and/or self-awareness. Qigong does have some exercises practiced like yoga on the ground, but curriculum really depends upon the teacher and intended participants. This curriculum is vast and holds many options and variations to help those that are injured, ill, disable and may have other limitations. The following graphics offer a window into what qigong exercises look like.

Knowledgeable and well experienced teachers of qigong and yoga will drill down into the details and subtle nuances of these practices. The development is in the details. Trying to learn these methods and the many specifics can be as easy or difficult as the practitioner cares to engage. However, one of the main benefits of these practices is that by occupying one's thoughts with physical details, the mind becomes more engaged with the body. This is where the true healing begins when the breathing frequency is deliberately slowed down, the nervous system adjusts the delicate blood chemistry which in turn positively affects organ function.

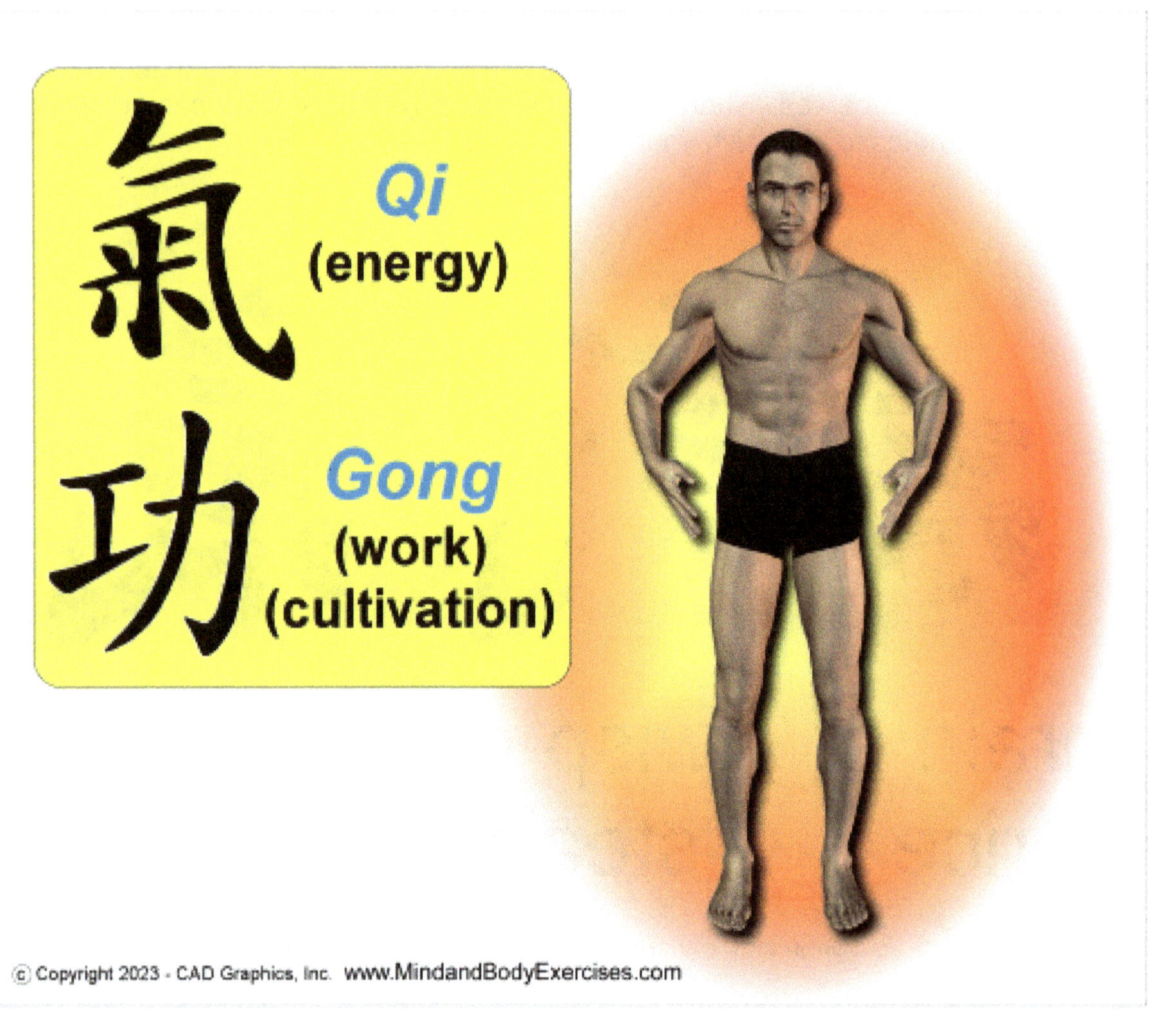

15. Qigong - Heal the Mind with the Body (a Detailed Description)

This is another post in my series of explaining qigong practices. Qi, Chi or Gi means air, energy or breath in Chinese and Korean. Gong or Kung means work. Qigong therefore translates to energy or breath work.

The human body is made up of bones, muscles, and organs amongst other components. Veins, arteries and capillaries carry blood and nutrients throughout to all of the systems and components. Additionally, 12 major energy meridians carry the body's energy. "lifeforce" also known as "qi". Ones qi is stored in the lower Dan Tien. Daily emotional imbalances accumulate tension and stress gradually affecting all of the body's systems. Each discomfort, nuisance, irritation or grudge continues to tighten and squeeze the flow of the life force. This is where "dis-ease" claims its foothold.

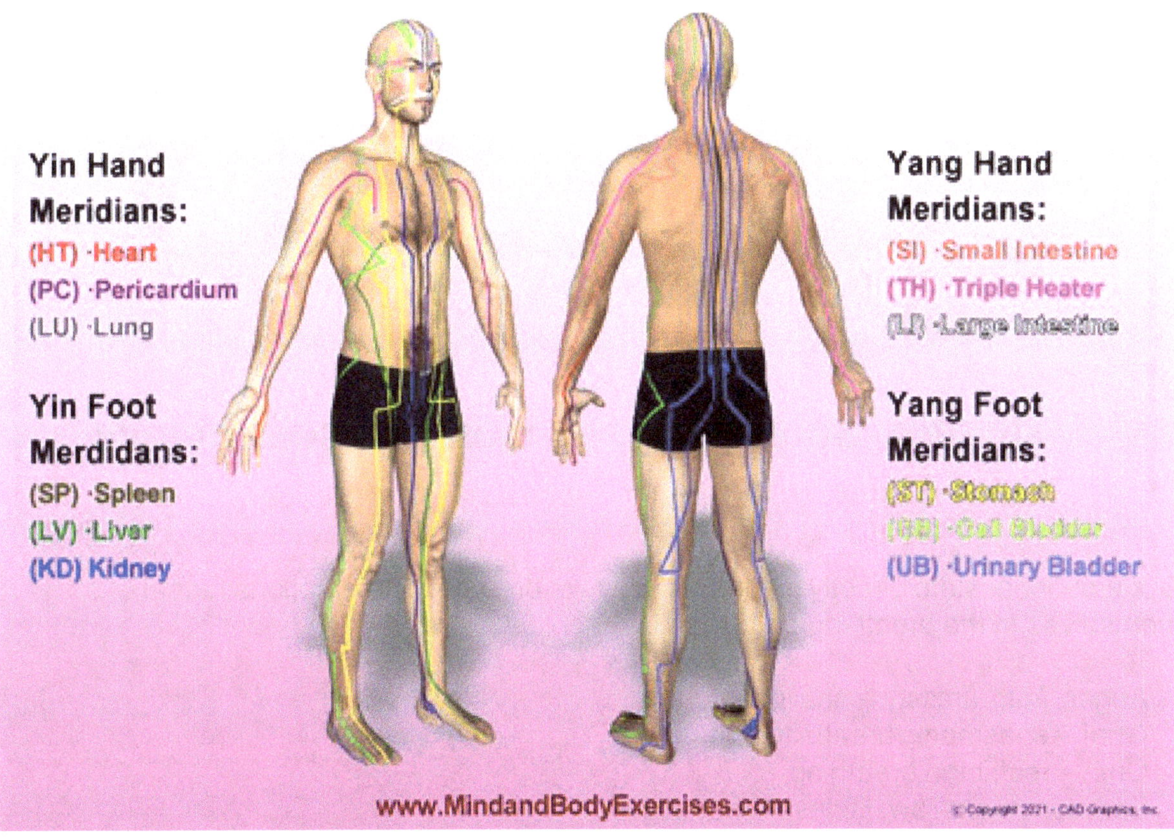

Qigong breathing exercises can adjust the brainwaves to the Alpha state, where the mind is relaxed and the body chemistry changes and promotes natural healing. Relaxing of the deep skeletal muscles and working outward as one tries to release tension accumulated within the muscles, organs and nerves. Whereas conventional physical exercise can deplete energy, Qi Gong helps to replenish your natural energy.

Similar to a sponge, the body absorbs positive as well as negative energy . Each emotion effects an internal organ. Qi Gong helps to balance the emotions:

Liver - anger, depression
Heart - excess of joy
Spleen - worry
Lung - grief
Kidney - fear

Healthy Sponge

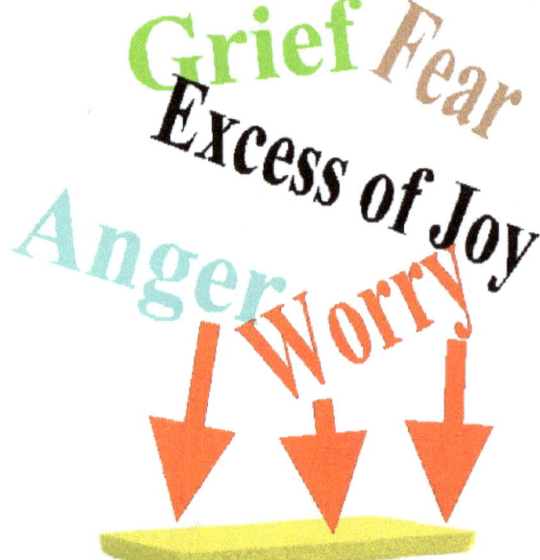

Compressed Sponge

Our emotional state directly influences how we breathe. The emotions reveal themselves in the breathing patterns:

Anger, fear, anxiety – shallow breaths
Grief – spasmodic breathing
Guilt – restricted breathing
Boredom – shallow, lifeless breathing
Sadness/depression – under breathing

Furthermore:
Dwelling in the past – can produce any of the above breathing patterns
Worrying about the future – can produce any of the above breathing patterns
Present in the moment – The goal here is clarity and self-awareness to slow and regulate the breath

Becoming present in the moment can happen in various ways such as:
1) Immediate trauma – Fear of injury or loss of life can put one into the moment quickly.

2) Practice of mindful exercises such as meditation, yoga, tai chi, qigong and other similar mind and body interactive practices.

3) Engaging in activities such as singing, painting, performing music, dancing, etc.

Qigong exercise can change brainwaves to the Alpha state:
Alpha – relaxed concentration, creative state
Beta – attentive, alert
Delta – unconscious
Theta – drowsy state of mind

Benefits of Qigong exercises:
Boosts the immune system
Reduce stress, anxiety, depression, mood swings
Lowers blood pressure
Increases the body's natural healing process
Lungs increase their capacity
Promotes better respiration and circulation
Enhanced self-awareness
Helps to change the body's chemistry for the better

Qigong utilizes regulated breathing, which calms emotions, which modulates the autonomic nervous system. This engages the parasympathetic nervous system that manages blood chemistry and relative hormones and neurotransmitters. Blood chemistry affects organ function either in a positive or negative manner.

The moment you change your perception, is the moment you rewrite the chemistry of your body. - Dr. Bruce Upton

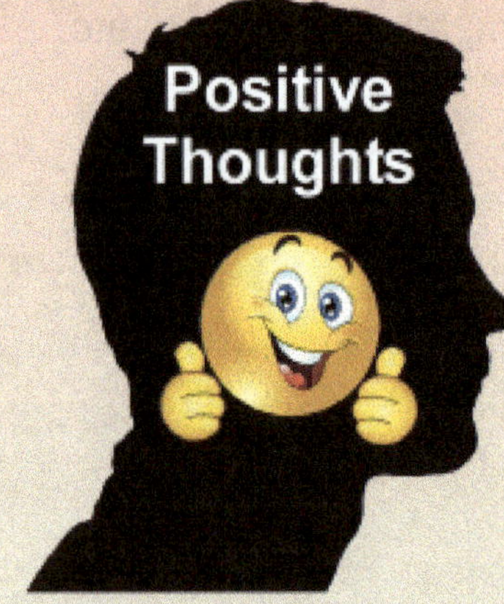

Bees Produce Honey

Bees Can Sting

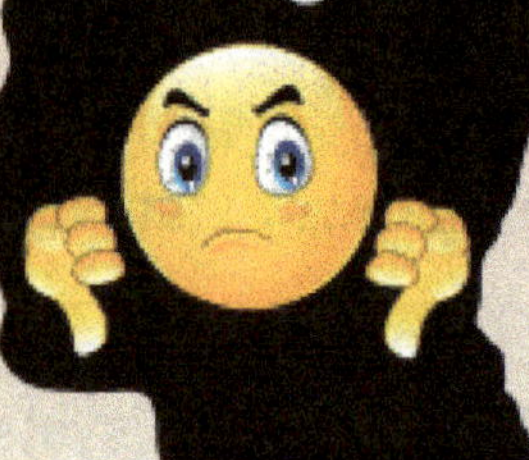

Half Full

Half Empty

"Happy Hormones"

Dopamine
The reward chemical
- celebrate small wins
- certain foods
- practicing self-care activities

Oxytocin
The love hormone
- hugging someone
- playing with pets
- socializing
- helping others
- hand holding

Serotonin
The mood stabilizer
- sun exposure
- exercise
- nature walks
- meditation

Endorphin
The pain killer
- laughter
- exercise
- listening to music
- essential oils

Get your daily DOSE of:

Dopamine
Oxytocin
Serotonin
Endorphin

"Stress Hormones"

Cortisol
The death hormone
- increase blood pressure
- counteracts insulin
- suppresses immune system
- increase sodium & water retention
- reduces bone formation

Adrenaline
The fight & flight hormone
- prepares body to handle difficult or danger situations
- persistent high levels can lead to anxiety, depression, heart disease, weight gain

Norepinephrine
The fight & flight hormone
- increases heart rate & blood pumping from the heart
- increases blood pressure
- break down fat & increase blood sugar levels to provide more energy to the body

www.MindandBodyExercises.com

Best Times:
- morning (calm, nature awakening)
- evenings (calm, tranquil)
- anytime (even a few minutes)

Best Locations to practice:
- outside and peaceful
- inside and uncluttered
- anywhere possible

Neutral, Horse-riding or "Wuji" Stance and Alignments

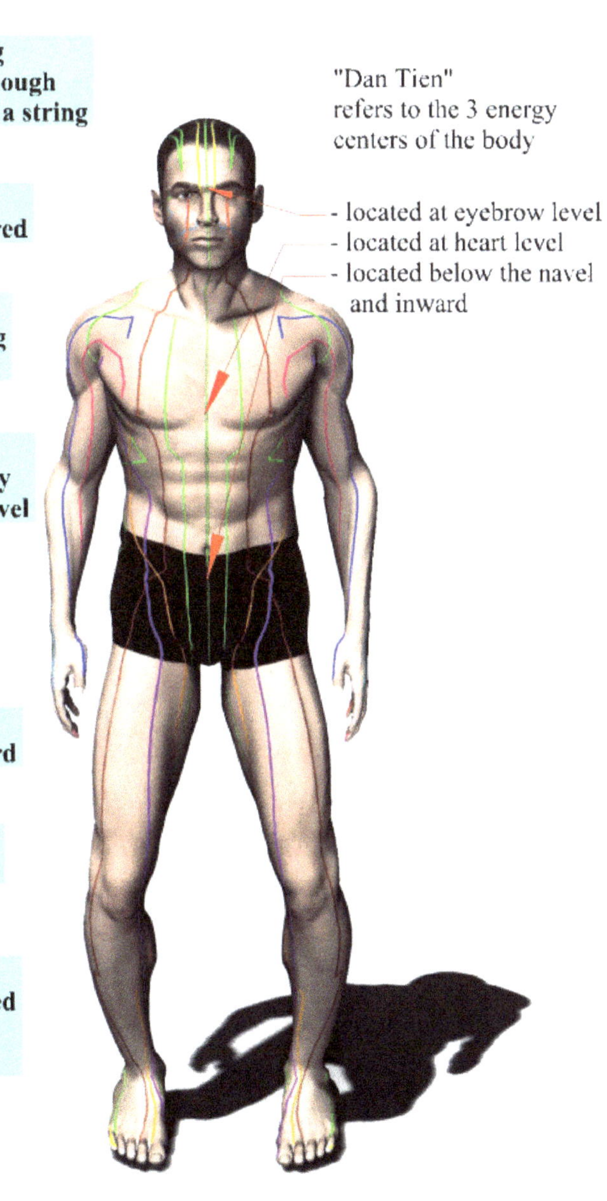

Basic Qigong exercise:

1) Stand, sit or lay in a position as shown to the right.

2) Try to align the body as listed in the steps on the previous page.

3) Inhale and exhale through the nose as the tongue gently touches the roof of the mouth behind the teeth.

4) Relax the forehead, eyebrows, eyelids, eyes, cheeks, lips and the jaw. close the mouth but don't clench your teeth.

5) Close the eyes to take away the distractions of what your eyes see.

6) Try to picture your body in your thought as you begin a scan from the top of your head working downward towards the toes.

7) As you think of the different parts of the body, try to imagine the deep skeletal muscles releasing from the bones as if they were melting or dissolving away.

8) Continue to become more self-aware of where you are holding tension within the body. As you exhale, try to release any tension in those areas by "dissolving" it away.

9) Follow your breath from the diaphragm as you till the lungs from bottom to top.

10) Let the stomach muscles pull inward as exhaling and bringing your thought back downward to just below the navel to the "Lower Dan Tien".

11) Continue this process as long or little as you choose, mindful that longer periods of time don't necessarily reflect increased benefits if not performed correctly. However, most benefits are arrived at over a period of time with consistent practice.

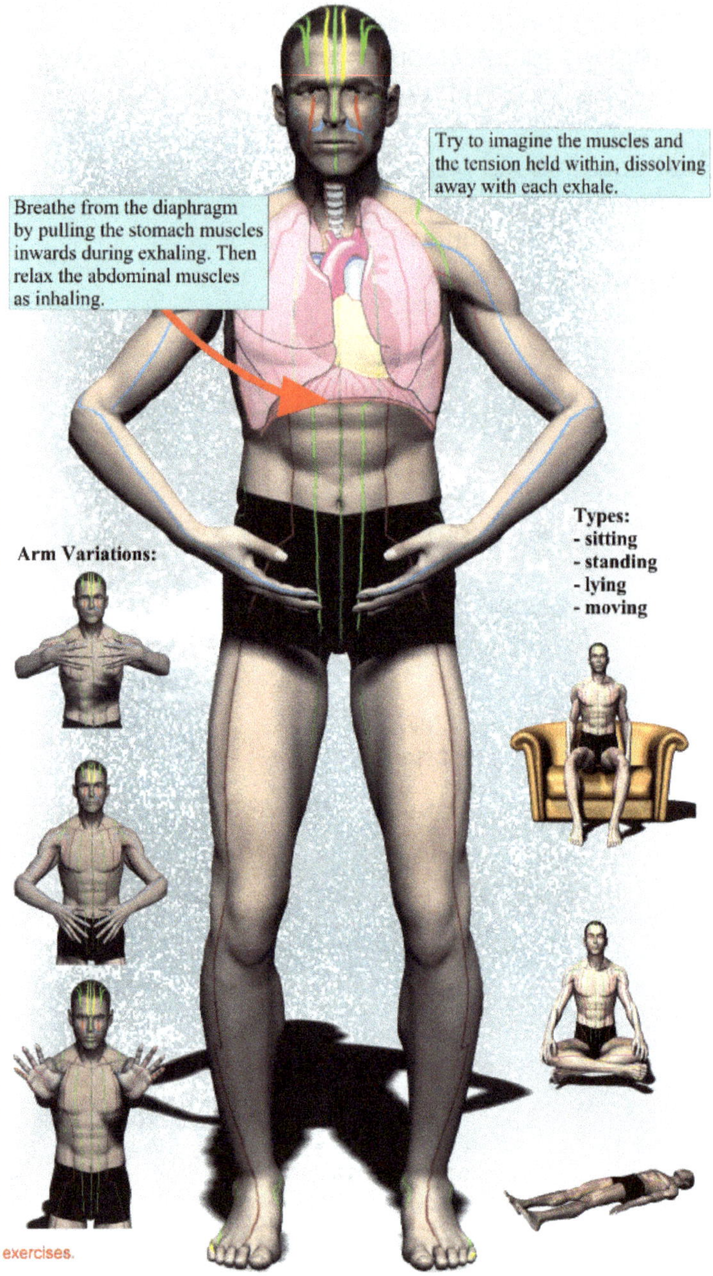

Find qualified teachers for actual instruction.
n a physician if uncertain of your physical abilities to perform such exercises.

Try to imagine the muscles and the tension held within, dissolving away with each exhale.

Breathe from the diaphragm by pulling the stomach muscles inwards during exhaling. Then relax the abdominal muscles as inhaling.

Arm Variations:

Types:
- sitting
- standing
- lying
- moving

Qigong practice is a solution to the current health care crisis, where we have seen a drastic increase in diabetes, obesity, depression, anxiety, stress, suicide and so many other mental and physically related health issues.

Would it not be wise to at least consider preventing these ailments in the first place rather than using questionable pharmaceuticals and therapies after the fact? Folks, the horse has been out of the barn for many decades now. If government leaders, medical professionals, school boards and parents were to actually promote and encourage physical exercise, good nutrition, meditation and self-responsibility we might have a much different looking nation. Plant good seeds, no?

Part V – Energy, Culture, and Philosophy

16. Chakras, Dan Tiens & The Hierarchy of Needs

Various theories exist as to how energy and thought manifest in physical form within and around the human body. These concepts seem new to Western culture, although other cultures have accepted their existence at least for many generations if not, thousands of years. Some modern personality theories have a close relationship with ancient philosophies (some may call these religions) of Taoism, Buddhism and Hinduism that have existed and been studied for thousands of years. There seems to me to be quite some overlap and maybe even borrowing from the ancients.

Abraham Maslow's Hierarchy of Needs also reflects similarities to the 7 chakras found in Buddhism and Hinduism. The 7 chakras or energy centers are thought to hold mental as well as physical aspects of human development. For example, the 1st chakra is the root chakra, similar to Maslow's basic needs of safety, survival, and primal instincts. The 7th chakra, also called the crown, corresponds to understanding, transcendence and enlightenment, similar to where Maslow's self-actualization where an individual struggles with morality and ethics. Again, these are familiar concepts and goals within other Eastern practices of philosophy and/or religion. Whether discussing chakras, dan tiens, energy meridians or the hierarchy of needs, all are intrinsically connected to our thoughts affecting our bodies, as well as our bodies affecting our thoughts.

Chakras
Coming from traditional Indian medicine, there exist 7 energy centers within the human body. These points are considered the focal points for the reception and transmission of energy. Some believe the chakras interact with the body's ductless endocrine glands and lymphatic system by feeding in positive energies and disposing of unwanted negative energies. Each chakra in your spinal column is believed to influence or direct bodily functions near its region of the spine.

Dan Tiens
There are 3 Dan Tien, or energy centers within the human body. The upper Dan Tien is located between the eyebrows and is associated with higher awareness. The middle Dan Tien is located near the center of the chest and affects the immune system by stimulating the heart and lungs. The lower Dan Tien is located just below the naval and affects the storage of energy in the kidneys.

Energy Meridians
There are 12 main medians and 8 other special meridians within the human body. Meridians are similar to electrical wires or nerves. They run from the top of the head to the tips of the toes and finger. Each meridian is associated with an internal organ. When there is a lack of flow or blockage within the meridians, health problems can arise. Through proper diet, exercises and lifestyle, it is possible to keep the chi flowing through the meridians.

Chakra Relationship to Hierarchy of Needs

Element	Energy Center	Chakra Name	Issues	Hierarchy of Needs (by Maslow)
Thought	7th	Crown	Understanding, Transcendence	SELF-ACTUALIZATION Morality, Creativity
Light	6th	Third Eye	Clarity, Wisdom, Intuition	AESTHETIC Beauty, harmony
Sound	5th	Throat	Expression, Communication	COGNITIVE Knowledge, Curiosity
Air	4th	Heart	Relationships, Love & devotion	ESTEEM Confidence, Achievement, Respect
Fire	3rd	Solar Plexus	Will, Power, Vitality, growth	BELONGING Love, Intimacy, Friendships
Water	2nd	Sacral	Joy, Sexuality, Emotions	SAFETY Health, Order, Stability
Earth	1st	Root	Physical Needs, Safety, Survival	PHYSICAL NEEDS food, sleep, sex, homeostasis

www.MindandBodyExercises.com

Chakra Correspondences

Energy Center	Name	Physical Location	Element	Issues	Right	Color	Note
1st	Root	Base of Spine	Earth	Physical Needs, Safety, Stability	To Have	Red	C
2nd	Sacral	Lower Abdomen	Water	Joy, Sexuality, Emotions	To Feel	Orange	D
3rd	Solar Plexus	Solar Plexus	Fire	Will, Power, Vitality	To Act	Yellow	E
4th	Heart	Heart	Air	Relationships, Love	To Love	Green	F
5th	Throat	Throat	Sound	Expression, Communication	To Speak	Blue	G
6th	Third Eye	Brow	Light	Clarity, Wisdom, Intuition	To See	Indigo	A
7th	Crown	Top of Head	Thought	Understanding, Transcendence	To Know	Violet	B

www.MindandBodyExercises.com

Energy Centers of the Human Body

www.MindandBodyExercises.com

Different schools of thought exist as to how energy exists within and around the human body. These concepts seem new to Western culture, although other cultures have accepted their existence at least for many generations if not, thousands of years.

Chakras

Coming from traditional Indian medicine, there exist 7 energy centers within the human body. These points are considered the focal points for the reception and transmission of energies. Some believe believe the chakras interact with the body's ductless endocrine glands and lymphatic system by feeding in positive energies and disposing of unwanted negative energies. Each chakra in your spinal column is believed to influence or direct bodily functions near its region of the spine.

Dan Tiens

There are 3 Dan Tien, or energy centers within the human body. The upper Dan Tien is located between the eyebrows and is associated with higher awareness. The middle Dan Tien is located near the center of the chest and effects he immune system by stimulating the heart and lungs. The lower Dan Tien is located just below the naval and effects the storage of energy in the kidneys.

Energy Meridians

There are 12 main medians and 8 other special meridians within the human body. Meridians are similar to electrical wires or nerves. They run from the top of the head to the tips of the toes and finger. Each meridian is associated with an internal organ. When there is a lack of flow or blockage within the meridians, health problems can arise. Through proper diet, exercises and life style, it is possible to keep the chi flowing through the meridians.

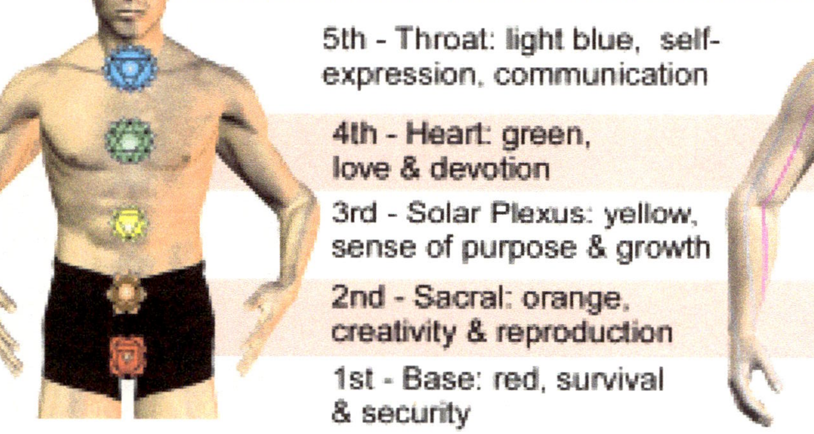

The 12 Primary Energy Meridians

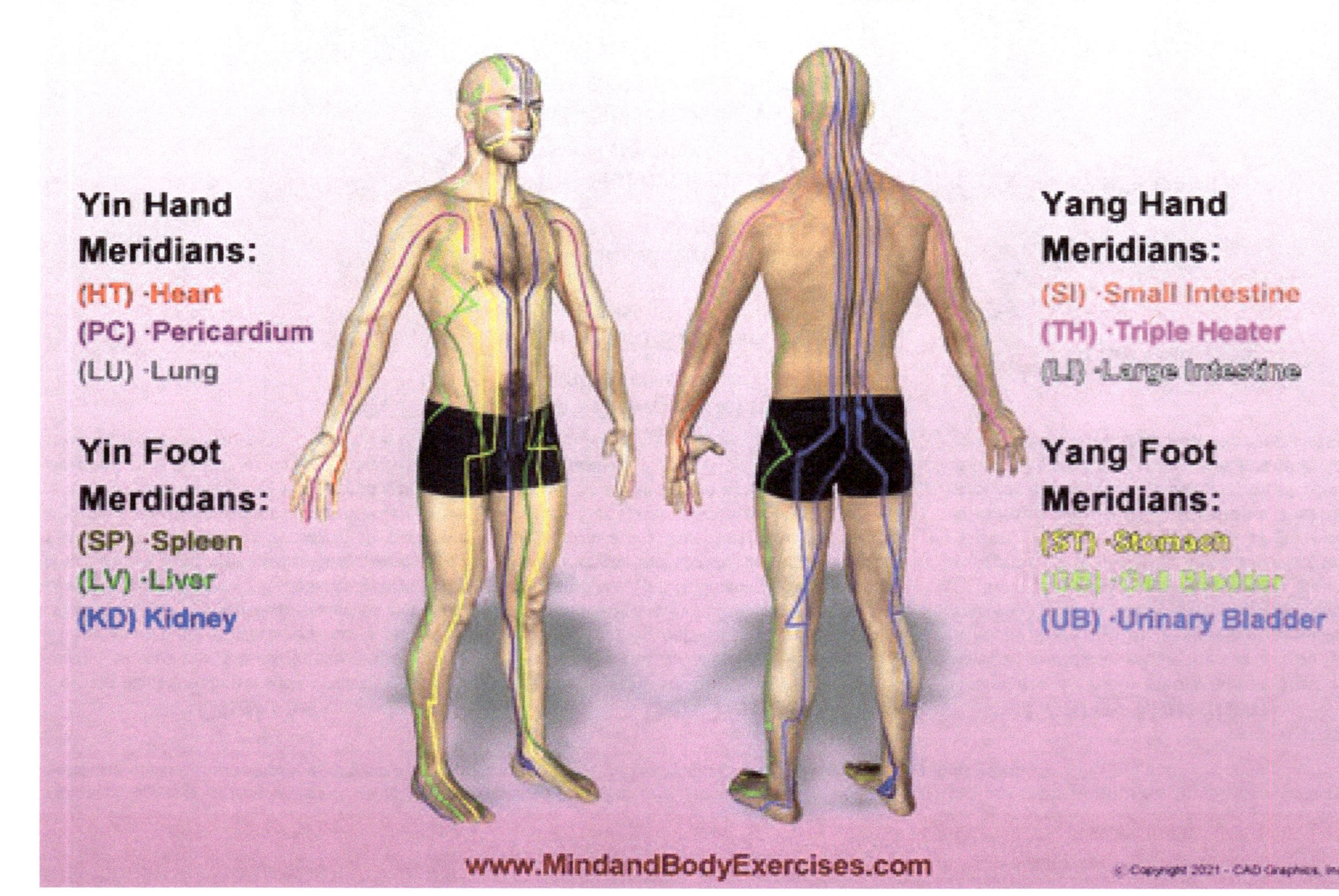

18. Sam Shim U Gye: Exploring Myth of Martial Multiplicity

The martial arts world has long held space for not only physically demonstrable technique but also oral teachings that border on the mystical. One such term that is rarely documented but occasionally referenced in specific martial circles is ***Sam Shim U Gye***. Roughly interpreted as "Three-Minded Five Principles" or "Three Mental States and Five Disciplines," this phrase suggests a layered understanding of human perception, psychological multiplicity, and strategic movement. Unlike somewhat known practices like *Kyung Gong Sul Bope, Qing Gong* (light body skill) or *Dim Mak* (death touch), *Sam Shim U Gye* remains mostly undocumented in formal Korean martial systems. Yet, within certain oral traditions, it is spoken of in association with the ability to move so swiftly or unpredictably that one appears to be in multiple places at once.

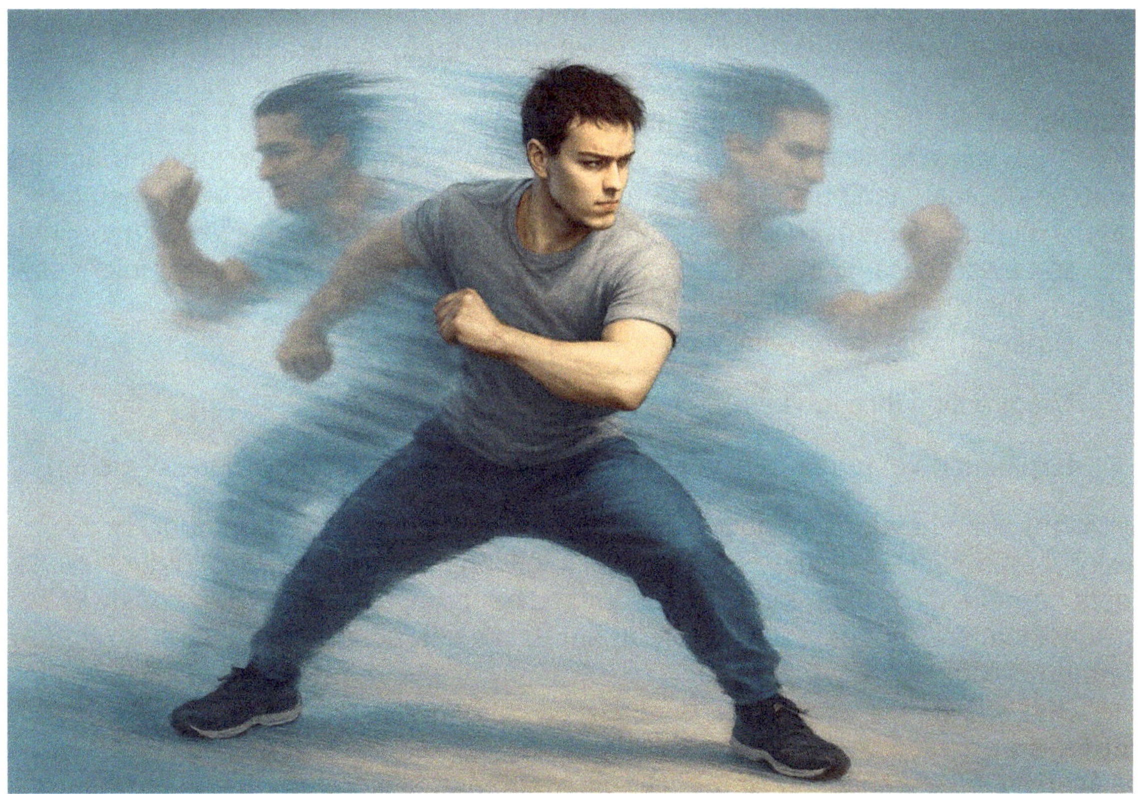

This essay aims to examine the term's potential meaning, its symbolic relationship to martial illusions of multiplicity, and its resonance with broader esoteric traditions such as *fenshen* from Daoist lore. While there is little scholarly reference to *Sam Shim U Gye*, analyzing its components and inferred application offers valuable insight into how martial legends and perceptual mastery intertwine.

Linguistic and Symbolic Deconstruction

A tentative breakdown of *Sam Shim U Gye* reveals a phrase built on classic East Asian symbolic logic:

- **Sam:** "Three"
- **Shim:** "Mind" or "Heart" (connoting consciousness, awareness, or intention)
- **U:** Possibly a linking particle; could also mean "space" or "again"
- **Gye:** Could denote "breath," "vital force," or "energy,"

Taken together, the phrase may imply a structured methodology of mental control, such as:

"Three Minds Merging or Projecting Energy", or even possibly
"The Three-Mind Energy Method."

In oral accounts, *Sam Shim U Gye* has been linked to the ability of a martial artist to move with such unpredictability, speed, or rhythm disruption that they appear to be multiplying themselves, a visual illusion often mistaken for supernatural ability.

Perceived Multiplicity and Martial Illusion
Rather than literal replication, *Sam Shim U Gye* may be better understood through the lens of perceptual manipulation. Human visual processing can be overwhelmed by sudden, rapid movement combined with environmental cues such as low light or limited peripheral awareness. Under these conditions, a highly trained practitioner might seem to "divide" their presence via:

- Broken rhythm and redirection
- Misdirection through layered footwork
- Exploitation of perceptual lag (e.g., saccadic masking, persistence of vision)

This aligns with the more formally attested Chinese concept of ***fenshen***, or "body division," found in Daoist texts like *Baopuzi* (Ge Hong, c. 320 CE). Ge Hong recounts adepts capable of creating multiple illusory bodies or appearing simultaneously in different locations, not as a physical feat, but as a spiritual or meditative realization (Campany, 2002).

Oral Tradition vs. Scholarly Canon
The scarcity of references to *Sam Shim U Gye* in martial literature raises an important distinction between documented tradition and oral transmission. Some martial teachings, particularly those tied to esoteric or family-based systems, were passed down verbally, often encoded in metaphoric or poetic language. In such cases, a term like *Sam Shim U Gye* might serve not as a technical formula but as a mnemonic device for internal principles: controlling one's mind, reading the opponent, and using deceptive motion to shape perception.

In modern application, this principle might be observed in elite-level athletes, such as boxers or mixed martial artists, who use feints and timing to "vanish" from the opponent's field of awareness, creating the illusion of multiple directions or unpredictable angles.

Comparative Frameworks: Qi Gong, Taoist Visualization, and Wuxia Myths
Sam Shim U Gye also echoes internal energy traditions where the mind is trained to "split" focus between different bodily centers or project awareness beyond the self. In certain ***neigong*** practices, advanced practitioners visualize "three fields" of awareness where the head, heart, and lower *dantian*, are simultaneously active. Similarly, in ***wuxia*** cinema (e.g., *Crouching Tiger, Hidden Dragon*), warriors are depicted leaping through trees or striking multiple foes with dazzling speed, mythical metaphors for an elite practitioner's fluid, multidimensional control of space. This myth-making often draws on the history of the Shaolin Monastery and its integration of martial discipline and spiritual cultivation (Shahar, 2008)

This symbolism doesn't imply literal multiplication but reflects an ideal of internal plurality and external coherence: being everywhere at once by being completely in tune with one's body, environment, and opponent.

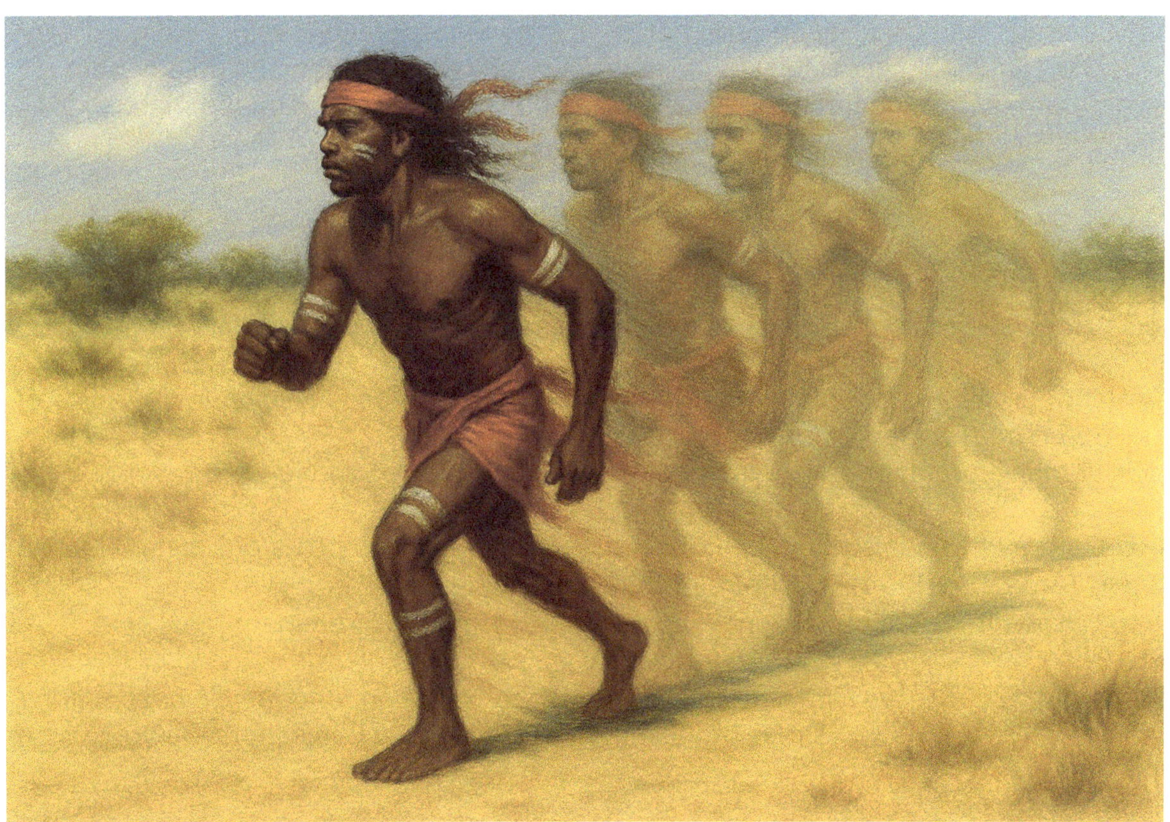

Though undocumented in formal literature, *Sam Shim U Gye* offers a compelling conceptual framework for understanding how martial artists manipulate perception through timing, positioning, and psychology. Its language evokes internal states of divided attention and strategic redirection, rather than mystical powers. When interpreted in tandem with Daoist *fenshen*, Aboriginal "shadow walking," and modern neurology, *Sam Shim U Gye* reveals itself as a metaphorical map of how disciplined minds and bodies can create illusions so powerful they border on the mythic.

Rather than dismissing such phrases as fantasy, we are invited to explore how martial artists throughout history have refined their craft, not only through physical conditioning, but through perception, awareness, and intention. In doing so, *Sam Shim U Gye* becomes less a supernatural claim and more a poetic blueprint for mastering complexity within stillness, motion, and mind.

Buyer Beware: Esoteric Claims and Modern Exploitation

In the pursuit of learning rare and esoteric methods such as *kyung gong sul bope*, *sam shim u gye*, or *dim mak,* aspiring students should exercise discernment. While historical legends, cultural folklore, and cinematic portrayals like *Crouching Tiger, Hidden Dragon* stir fascination with superhuman potential, they also invite opportunism. There are individuals and groups who present these elusive skills as secrets they alone have mastered, often demanding steep financial or personal commitments. Without empirical validation or lineage-based verification, such claims can mislead the hopeful and exploit the vulnerable. As Carl Sagan aptly noted, *"extraordinary claims require extraordinary evidence."* Caution, critical thinking, and humility are vital companions on any path toward human development, especially when the line between myth and mastery is intentionally blurred.

References

Campany, R. F. (2002). *To Live as Long as Heaven and Earth: A Translation and Study of Ge Hong's Traditions of Divine Transcendents*. University of California Press.

Ge Hong. (trans. Ware, J. R.). (1966). *Alchemy, Medicine and Religion in the China of A.D. 320: The Nei Pien of Ko Hung*. Dover Publications. https://archive.org/details/alchemymediciner00ware/page/n5/mode/2up

HKU Centre of Buddhist Studies. (2024, June 19). The Biographies of Eminent Monks 高僧傳 (Free eBook) - HKU Centre of Buddhist Studies. https://www.buddhism.hku.hk/publication-post/biographies-of-eminent-monks/

Shahar, M. (2008). *The Shaolin Monastery: History, Religion, and the Chinese Martial Arts*. University of Hawai'i Press. https://archive.org/details/shaolinmonastery0000shah

19. Taoism Viewed as a Philosophy, Vitalizing or Religious

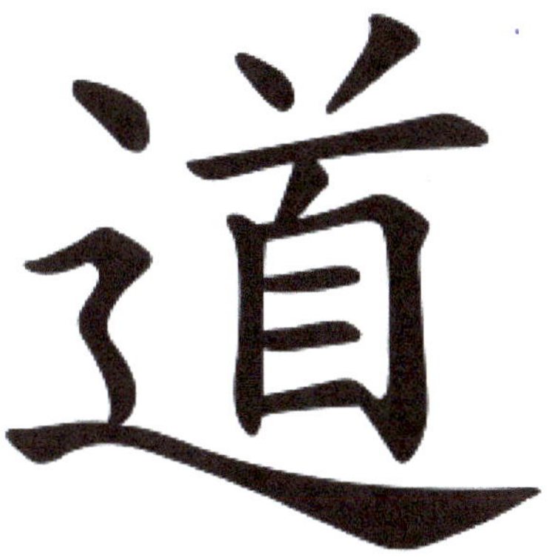

The Chinese character for *"the Tao"*

Taoism or Daoism is based upon the concept of the *Tao (or Dao)* and its literal meaning of the *path*, or *way*. The Tao is the main principle of Taoism, where the Tao is seen as the natural order of the universe. This understanding of the universe and all-encompassing things within whether alive or inanimate cannot be defined in mere words but rather become known through actual living experience in everyday beings (Smith, 2009).

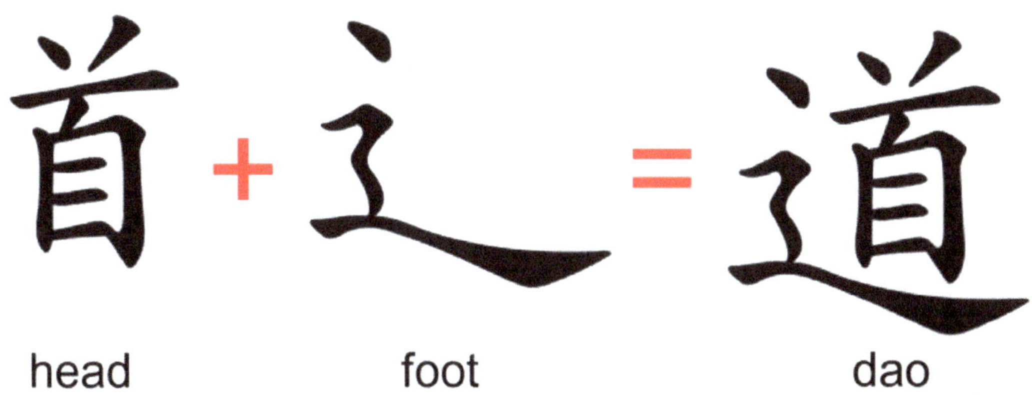

Dao or Tao, means "the way".

The Taoist individual becomes more reliant upon their own intuition in order to understand the potential for their own individual wisdom. The universe came into being with us together; with us, all things are one. The Tao is simply inconceivable, and therefore it is useless to say another word about it. Intuitively, we know there is a dimension of ourselves and of nature that eludes us because it is too close, too general, and too all-embracing to be singled out as a particular object. This dimension is the ground of all the astonishing forms and experiences of which we are aware. Because we are aware, it cannot be unconscious, although we are not conscious of it as an external thing. We can give it a name but cannot make any definitive statement about it. The only way of apprehending it is by watching the process and patterns of nature and by the meditative discipline of allowing our minds to become quiet, to have a vivid awareness of "what is" without verbal comment.

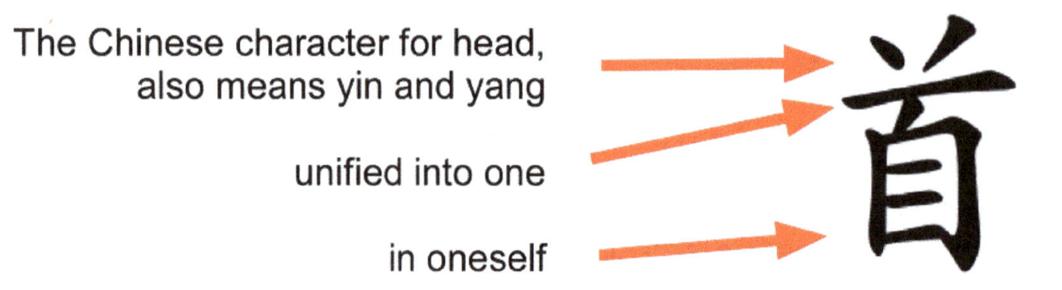

Chinese culture and its views on religion have evolved over many centuries with Confucianism, Taoism, and Buddhism being considered the "three pillars" of ancient Chinese society (National Geographic Society, 2022). Consequently, most Chinese people have practiced Confucianism in their ethics and public life, Taoism in their private life and hygiene, and Buddhism at the time of death, along with shamanistic folk religion also added in along the way. "Every Chinese wears a Confucian hat, Taoist robes, and Buddhist sandals" (Smith, 2009).

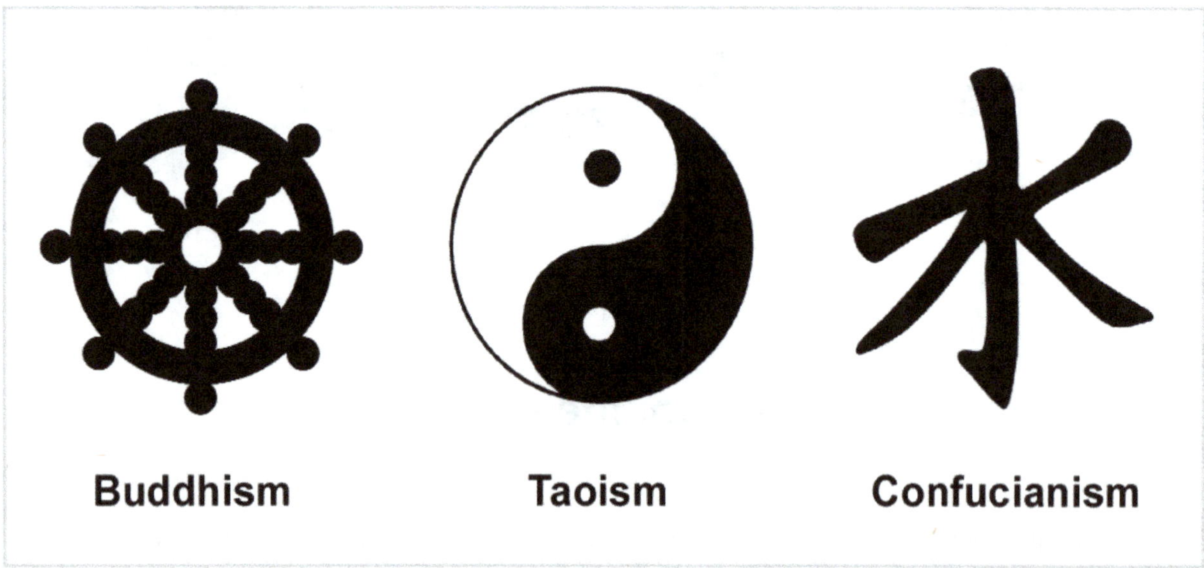

There are 3 main types of Taoism. The first type is referred to as philosophical Taoism, where it is essentially a frame of mind, where the goal is to conserve one's *te* or power, by expending it efficiently. This type of Taoism holds the main concept of *wu wei*, meaning "inaction" but in Taoism means pure effectiveness. Wu wei is an action in which the individual strives to minimize conflict in relationships and be in harmony with nature (Smith, 2009). This concept more simply stated would be to learn to "go with the flow". Attempting to exist in opposition to the Tao, one will eventually be consumed by it. Striving to live in harmony with the Tao or more specifically wu wei, will benefit from this relationship. Living more in harmony with the Tao can be often seen as being more out in the world and nature to experience its gifts while living a life interacting with nature as well as with others.

A second type of Taoism is "vitalizing" where practitioners strive to maximize their life force, also called *qi* or *chi*. These adepts worked with their minds, matter, and physical movement, to increase their life force (Smith, 2009). Some may find this branch of Taoism as more unusual or unfamiliar as Huston Smith called it a "vitality cult" (Smith, 2009). Most belief systems and/or religions are based upon the unknown, mysteries, and unconfirmed facts. To the uninformed, what is considered one person's religion may very well be another person's cult.

A third type of Taoism was influenced by Buddhism, being that of Religious Taoism. Here the actions of psychics, free-lance soothsayers, shamans, and faith healers who may have come by their powers naturally, religious Taoism institutionalized these activities (Smith, 2009). Religious Taoism appears as a crude superstition to the uneducated. At the time of Smith's observation, science knew little of what energy is, how it proceeds, or the means by which it can be utilized (Smith, 2009). However, currently, we do know about faith healing engaging energies, including faith in oneself. Placebos are now known and proven to have various healing effects mentally, physically, and/or spiritually.

I have had much firsthand experience with all 3 of these types of Taoism along with Buddhism and Confucianism, as a philosophical lifestyle, as my martial arts and qigong lineages are deeply rooted within these belief systems. I did not priorly nor formally study any of these philosophies but rather lived with them in my life. I see the concepts and principles found within these philosophies as being highly relevant to my everyday routine. I was raised within the Christian Church and more specifically the Lutheran and Disciples of Christ branches. Taoism does not oppose nor contradict these Christian faiths but rather supports morals and ethics found in many other religions.

The Taoist concept of *yin* and *yang*, where harmony and balance coexist, contrast and relativity are seen in all things in life and nature. Yin and yang ultimately affect all aspects of life in health, relationships, business, and even other religions in various other aspects. Yin and yang are much more than simply the contrast between dark and light. The symbol for this concept depicts cause and effect, ebb and flow, and other manifestations of harmony, and is known as the *Tajitu.* The symbol actually has more components than just the 2 fish-shaped halves. The complete circle itself consists of the two halves, plus the small dots of contrast found in each half, and lastly, the line that divides the two halves. These dots remind us that nothing is truly black or white, or absolute. The fine line resting between the two opposing halves may be viewed as the gray area that we sometimes find ourselves navigating when striving to balance our decisions. Decisions between what we perceive as true, right, or correct for whatever situation and circumstances relate to any particular time and place. What is seen as correct yesterday may not be so today; appropriate for one, may not be for another. These components collectively represent the ever-changing relationship of all of these various pieces and parts that make up the whole.

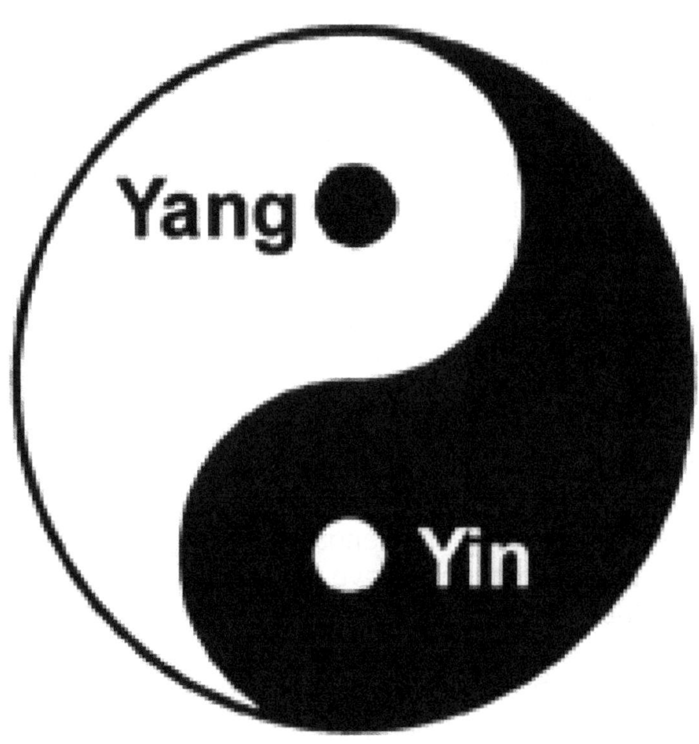

Meaning of the Yin-Yang Symbol

The yin and yang symbol or taijitu, relates to the day and night association of yin and yang. Supposedly the ancients plotted a graph made up of six concentrically larger rings. In the center was anchored an 8-foot high pole that measured the shadow cast by the sun throughout the seasons. Then they colored in where the shade landed and where there was none. When looked at from above, the graph showed a picture that resembles the yin and yang symbol but without the two dots on either side. From here the concept of balance and its relationship to the seasons and nature was conceived.

The yin-yang symbol has been long known to represent balance and harmony. However, some choose to label it as a religious symbol for Daoism which many consider more of a philosophy. The martial arts of tai chi uses this symbol and concept as a foundation to understanding of the flow of energy within the human body.

Summer Solstice
Autumn
Autumnal Equinox
Summer
YANG
YIN
Winter
Vernal Equinox
Spring
Winter Solstice

The Five Aspects of Yin and Yang

The 5 Aspects of yin and yang complement and balance each other via these aspects, which define the relationship between each.

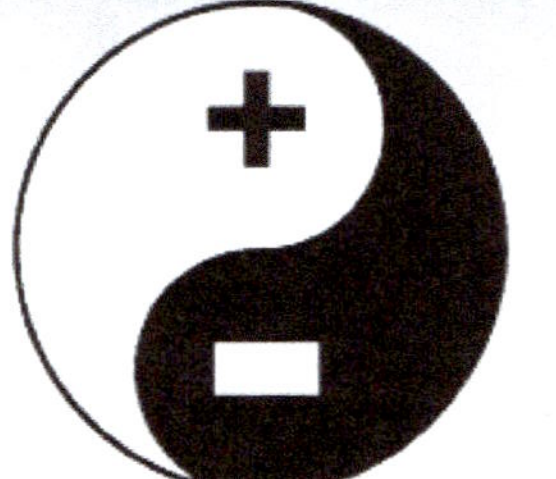

1) Opposition

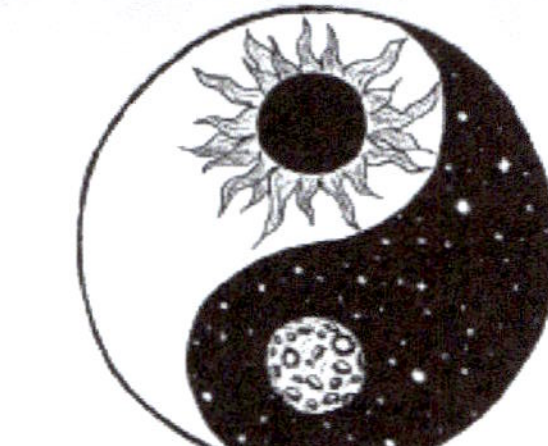

2) Interdependence

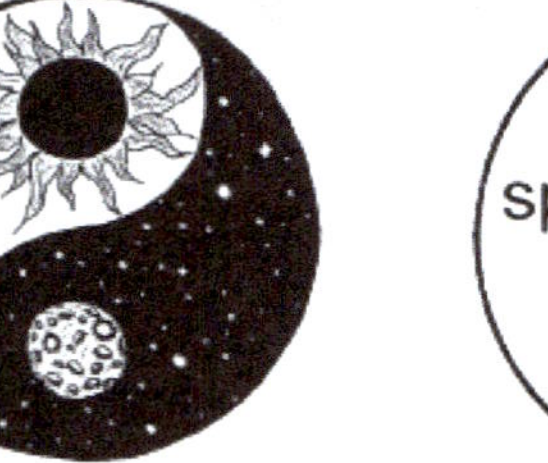

3) Mutual Consuming -Increasing

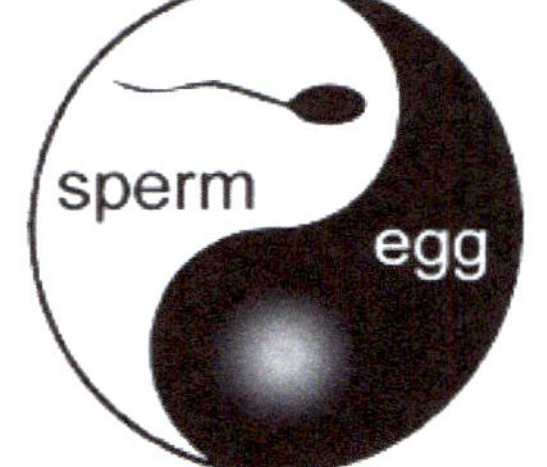

4) Mutual Transforming

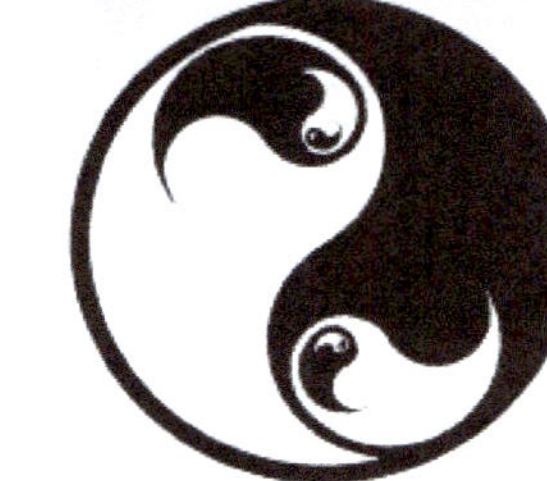

5) Infinite Divisibility

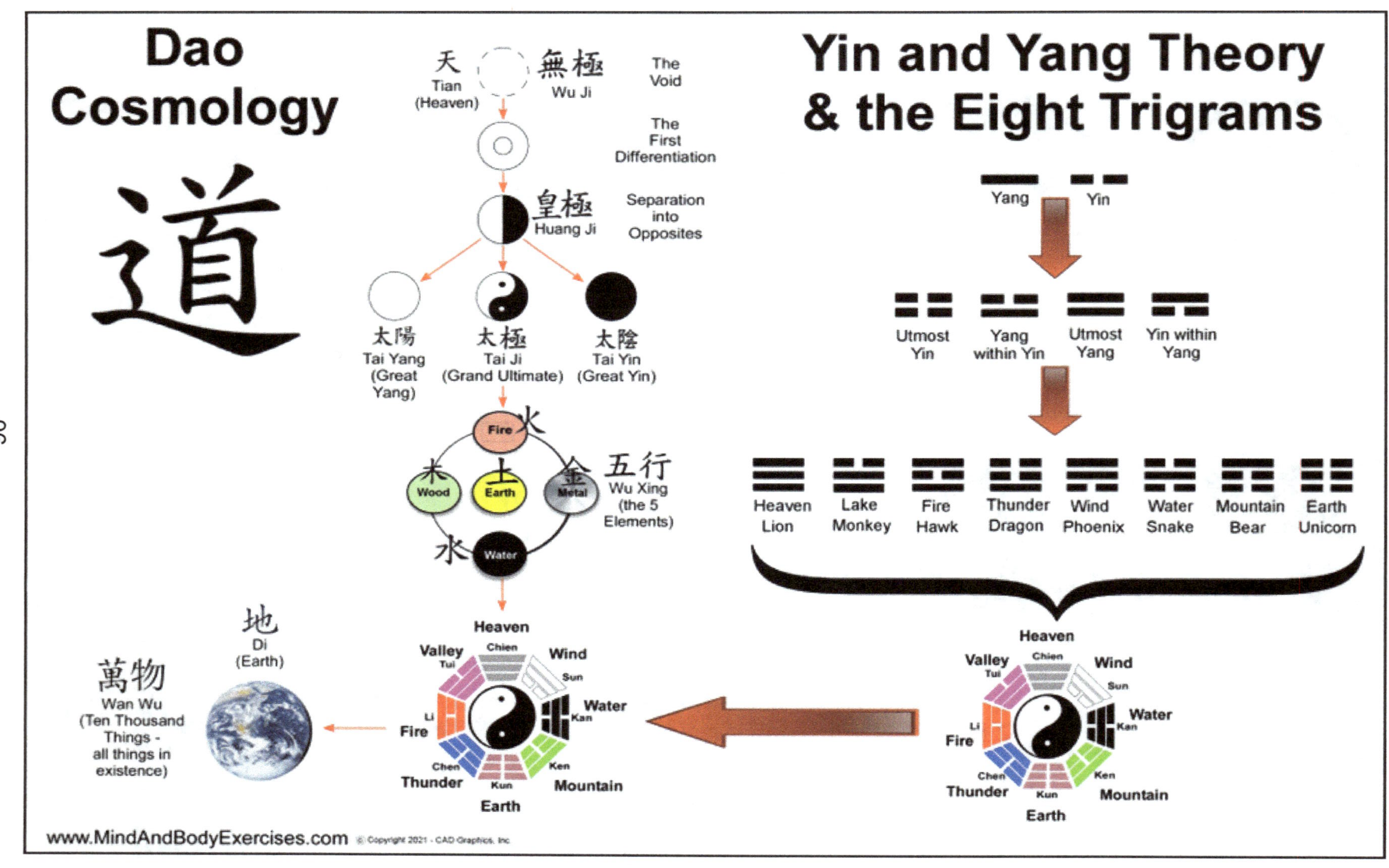

Dao Cosmology
道
天
Tian
(Heaven)
無極
Wu Ji
The Void
The First Differentiation
皇極
Huang Ji
Separation into Opposites
太陽
Tai Yang
(Great Yang)
太極
Tai Ji
(Grand Ultimate)
太陰
Tai Yin
(Great Yin)
火 Fire
木 Wood
土 Earth
金 Metal
水 Water
五行
Wu Xing
(the 5 Elements)
Heaven
Chien
Wind
Sun
Water
Kan
Ken
Mountain
Kun
Earth
Chen
Thunder
Li
Fire
Tui
Valley
地
Di
(Earth)
萬物
Wan Wu
(Ten Thousand Things - all things in existence)
Yin and Yang Theory & the Eight Trigrams
Yang
Yin
Utmost Yin
Yang within Yin
Utmost Yang
Yin within Yang
Heaven Lion
Lake Monkey
Fire Hawk
Thunder Dragon
Wind Phoenix
Water Snake
Mountain Bear
Earth Unicorn
Heaven
Chien
Wind
Sun
Water
Kan
Ken
Mountain
Kun
Earth
Chen
Thunder
Li
Fire
Tui
Valley
www.MindAndBodyExercises.com
© Copyright 2021 - CAD Graphics, Inc

Taoism does explain the creation of the Universe and what exists within it. The Tao transformed from the nothingness or *Wuji,* to yin and yang, then further into the 5 Elements or *Wuxing*, then to the 8 trigrams or *Bagua,* and eventually into the Ten Thousand Things. Some people may see these concepts as religious, while others may interpret as philosophy and maybe even others will see these ideas as a science of the universe.

The I Ching, a Taoist philosophical text written by Fu Xi around 1300 BCE, addresses 64 phases in that we go through in the process of becoming a human being (Hon, 2019). Through these phases, one can evolve from basically being unconscious to hopefully conscious, from an inferior to a superior human being. It actually takes considerable effort and time to become what we consider human. We are born basically like any other animal and more specifically a mammal, but with the potential abilities to learn to communicate and reason.

Upper trigram >> Lower trigram vv	Ch'ien	Chen	K'an	Kên	K'un	Sun	Li	Tui
Ch'ien	1	34	5	26	11	9	14	43
Chen	25	51	3	27	24	42	21	17
K'an	6	40	29	4	7	59	64	47
Kên	33	62	39	52	15	53	56	31
K'un	12	16	8	23	2	20	35	45
Sun	44	32	48	18	46	57	50	28
Li	13	55	63	22	36	37	30	49
Tui	10	54	60	41	19	61	38	58

Hexagrams of the I Ching

There is a fundamental belief within Taoism, that we are not born with the wisdom of being "correct" but rather we are born and begin to be "true" in our perceptions, words, and actions. For example, a child cries because they are hungry, expressing their true feelings of hunger pangs in their stomach. Later in life, that same child will learn that the correct way to express oneself may be to ask for food verbally.

We are usually not born as balanced or enlightened human beings. Humans are not intrinsically born as what we often label as "good". Our nature is seemingly good as an innocent little human being but basically, we are born as an animal with no inherent skill to survive physically or socially. Unguided children will not feed, clothe or potty-train themselves. If you look at any young child not nurtured, guided, or refined by a parent or mentor of that child, that child will instinctively do whatever they please until they meet with resistance. The child is not inherently "bad" but rather has instinctive behavior, similar to that of a little animal not knowing of boundaries or refinement. If the parent doesn't accept this duty of actual parenting, the child may eventually grow into an adult who spends their whole life behaving like an animal. If the parent does not take the time to give their child life direction by teaching with words and actions rooted in principle and love, that child will become a human being in physical form, while remaining an animal in their consciousness and relative actions.

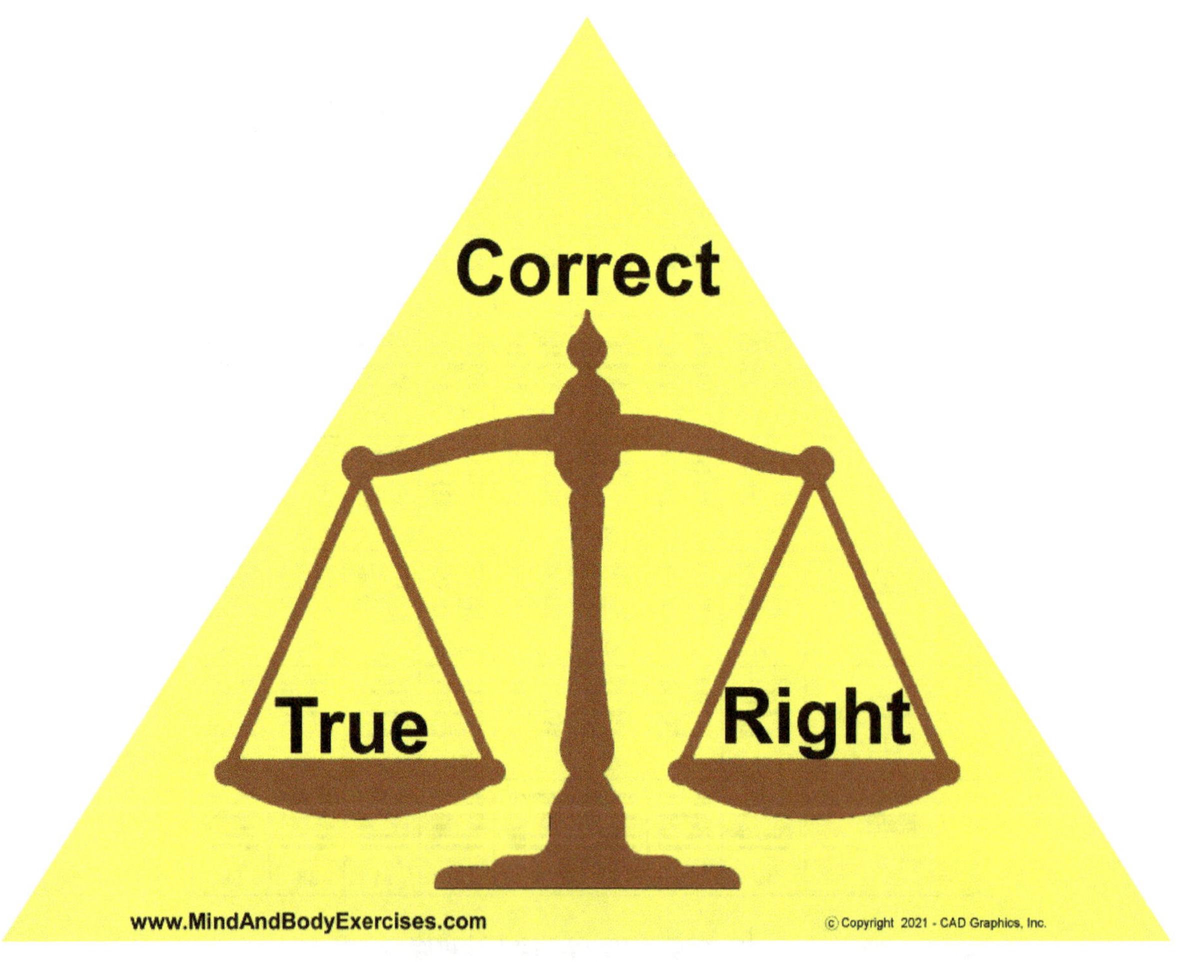

Some belief systems or philosophic schools of thought believe that we have to earn our human potential beyond that of being an animal. We are born into a particular set of circumstances or actions of cause and effect, known as *karma*, in Hinduism, Buddhism, and Taoism. Even before we arrive in the physical form of a zygote, embryo, or fetus, there is a belief structure that we already made an agreement based upon our karma, of what kind of resources one will come into this world with and relative life from these resources. These may include time and place of birth, physical or mental traits, ethnicity, status, and other cultural variables. Hopefully, the individual earned good karma in their past life because that affects where and to who they are born into.

Karma doesn't mean something that drops upon you from somewhere, Karma means your action, it's your making, it's your doing.

- Sadhguru

The first phase of life is childhood from birth to age 8, which is considered as Spring and is highly related to one's past karma. The individual child has very little control over their own current karma at this age, relying almost entirely upon where they were born and who their parents are. The order of the next phases of life would be Summer (ages 8-33), Late Summer (ages 33-58), Fall (ages 58-83), and Winter (ages 83-108). These phases of the year correspond accordingly with the 5 Element Theory or Wuxing (Wuxing, Internet Encyclopedia of Philosophy, n.d.), and the mental and physical changes we experience throughout our whole cycle of one lifetime.

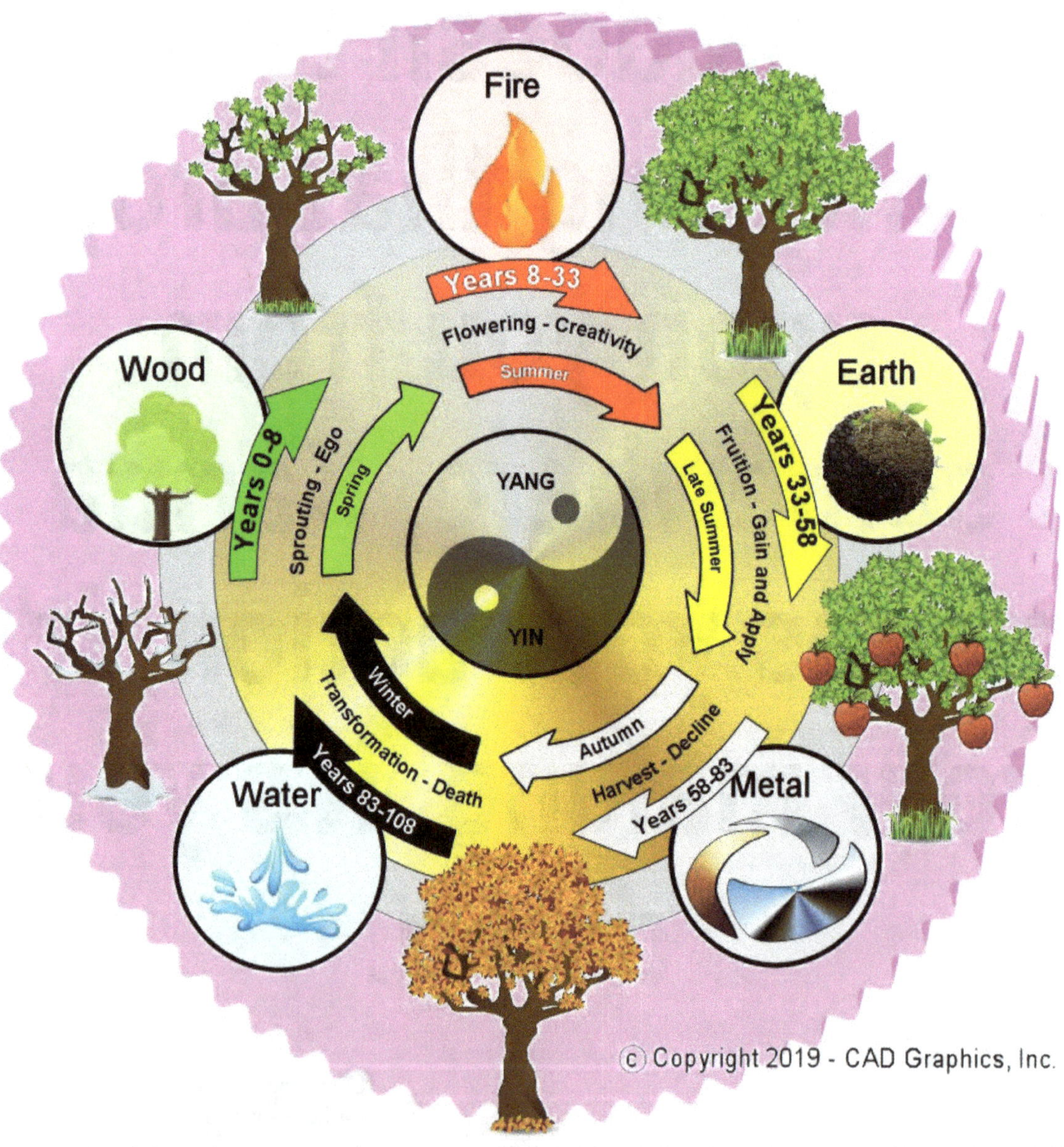

After the initial spring phase of childhood and into young adulthood or summer, the individual begins to work on choosing whether or not they are going to go through life in a state of unconscious suffering or go through life evolving as a conscious human being. Life is a challenge or struggle, and we all experience this struggle differently. The struggle never ends as we strive to become more human until we can no longer. Similar to standing upright on two feet, we always have a struggle to work and exert effort to stay standing. As soon as we stop working on standing, we fall. Consequently, there is this constant struggle to become more human or to use other labels such as self-realization or self-mastery. Realization in this context may be defined as having an advanced understanding of the interrelationship of their mind, body, and consciousness.

Self-cultivation is another appropriate term, as we ourselves are actually the garden that needs constant tending. Some among us may have started on this path decades long ago, trying to navigate within this lifestyle and path of self-cultivation. Some are considered spiritual teachers or leaders. They are not done yet, as we are never truly done as far as this physical life is concerned. If life is a constant struggle, the concept we have to accept is that no one is entitled to anything. If we truly want to change our reality, we need to realize that no one is going to change it for us. Not our friends, family, boss, government, or anyone other than ourselves. The universe and nature offer no entitlements that are going to change our individual reality. It starts with us taking ownership and responsibility to change our own set of circumstances and actions (karma) whether good or bad. If we look at our situations or circumstances as being someone else's fault or responsibility, we have lost control over our own life and our own potential outcomes. Ultimately, we may realize that we allow others the power to manage our lives until we choose to change this reality, as we alone choose to make ourselves good or make ourselves bad.

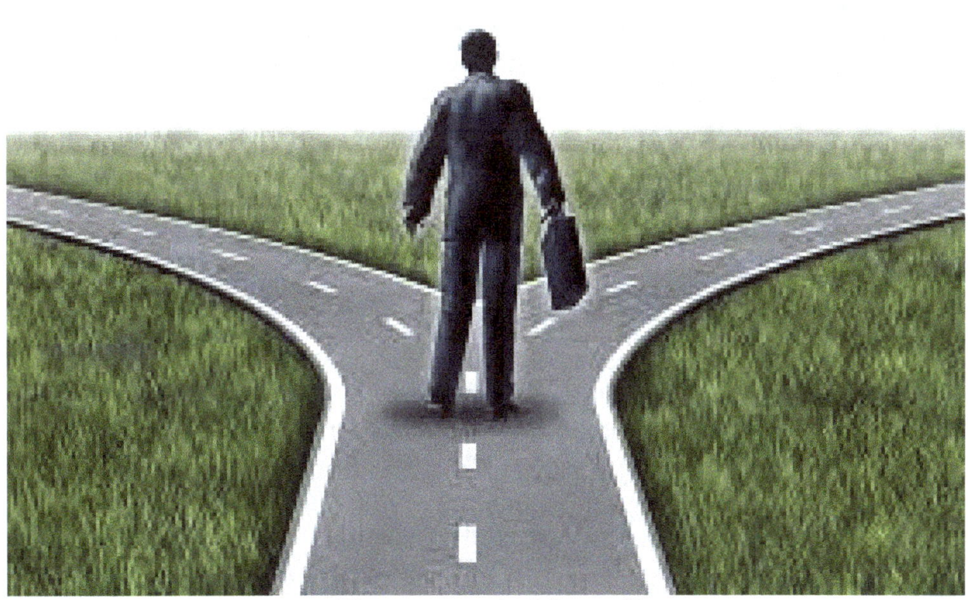

The concept of freewill

We have no true freedom if we are subject to the will of others. Self-cultivation is about taking total ownership of our own life and its direction. We have this choice every minute of every day, until death. Ancient and time-proven safe and effective methods of mind and body practices rooted in Buddhism and Taoism, such as yoga, tai chi, qigong, and other methods, offer ways to build character, strength, and self-discipline. Within some belief systems, these practices can affect one's karma. By regular and consistent execution in maintaining a particular posture or stance, despite the physical discomfort in doing so, the individual develops the fundamentals of self-discipline. These practices offer a very deliberate equation or recipe, to achieve self-cultivation. Self-cultivation cannot be achieved by luck or chance. Similar to traveling to a specific destination, one cannot easily reach their target by chance, without a map or sense of direction. Religions of Hinduism offer the *Yamas* and *Niyamas* whereas Christianity holds the 10 Commandments as guidance or maps of direction. Buddhism has the philosophy of the Eightfold Path and Islam has their 5 Pillars. The philosophy of Taoism has a similar guide in its own Eight-step Path.

This Eight-step Path of Taoism is where I will focus some attention. This path of processes is a map or recipe of insights that may lead to experiences in varying levels of evolution of our own consciousness. This recipe is rooted in the understanding that our life is basically a continuous yearly journey around the sun where we all go through the yearly cycles of the climatic seasons. The climate appears very random to us as children, where we see sun and rain for a while and then a time later of wind and snow. Until we are taught that there is a deliberate repeating cycle, this change in our surroundings, environment and relative weather patterns seems to be so random. When the child knowingly experiences a second or third year of the season changes, the climate becomes less confusing and actually more predictable. Similarly, the steps or cycles of the Eight-step Path may appear at first to be somewhat random but are quite deliberate.

The first step may be the most difficult, which is to truly see oneself in the highest expression of their humanness. The Sanskrit word of *namaste,* meaning of "may the divine in me see the divine in you". The challenge here is that in most cases, the individual cannot see the divine in others because they cannot see it first in themselves. This highly important component is in the reflection of actually looking inside of yourself. Often this step is most uncomfortable, where the individual is venturing outside of their comfort zone in order to go through the humility of seeing themselves in a less-than-perfect perspective. This is where methods of sitting, standing, and moving practices within yoga, qigong, tai chi, and others can offer these self-awareness reflections, in addition to their mere basic physical benefits of Westernized glorified stretching and breathing exercises. Beyond just exercising the body, these somewhat gentle methods can require the practitioner to become aware of their various aspects of weaknesses in their postural alignments, coordination, balance, and other facets of their self-awareness like breath and heart rate. Observing and becoming aware of our physical body is the gateway into becoming more aware of our complex thoughts and emotions.

The 8-Step Path to Achieve the Best Version of You

www.MindAndBodyExercises.com

A long-understood method of achieving harmony between one's mind, body and spirit, is this 8-Step Path. It has its origin in the ancient Chinese philosophy of Daoism but is highly relative to modern culture. The figure "8" is important to understand that as the infinity circle, there is no beginning nor end to entering into this process. It is a journey of self-awareness that can be entered into at any point throughout one's lifetime. Life is a challenge, and so is staying on this path of self-improvement. The reward is at the end of one's journey, knowing that they have pursued a meaningful life with direction and purpose.

1 Learning to Know Your "True Self"

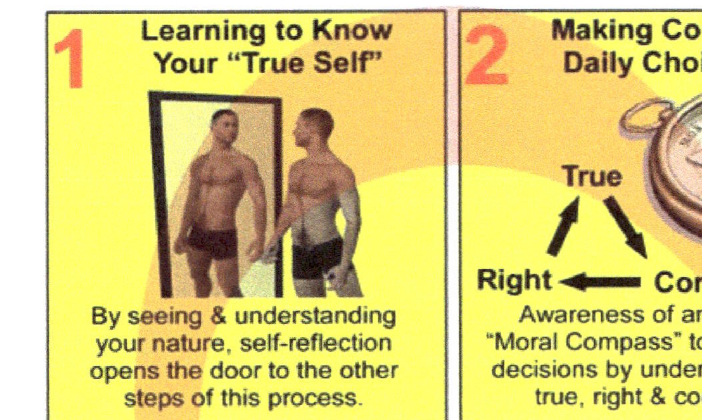

By seeing & understanding your nature, self-reflection opens the door to the other steps of this process.

2 Making Correct Daily Choices

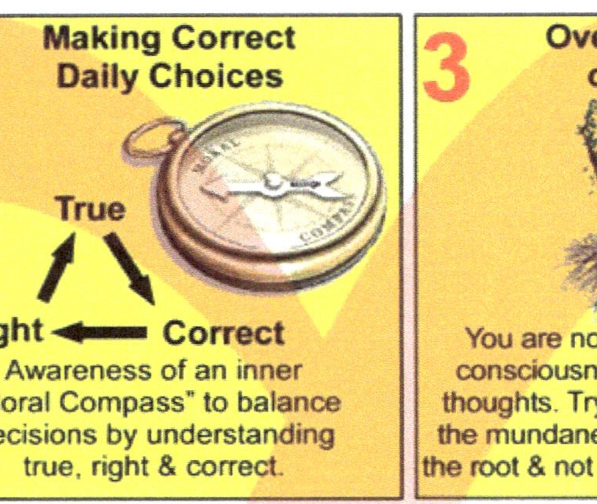

Awareness of an inner "Moral Compass" to balance decisions by understanding true, right & correct.

3 Overcome Delusion of Your Thoughts & Ideas

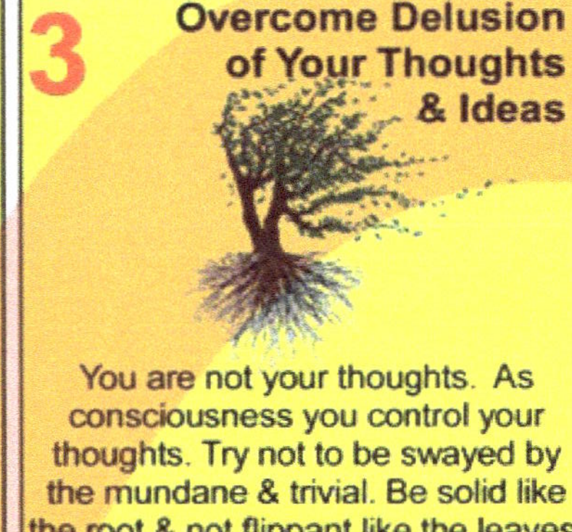

You are not your thoughts. As consciousness you control your thoughts. Try not to be swayed by the mundane & trivial. Be solid like the root & not flippant like the leaves.

4 Cultivate Good Seeds to Pass On

Realize that you have a higher purpose beyond gaining material wealth and status. Be the light at the end of the tunnel.

5 Attain Honor

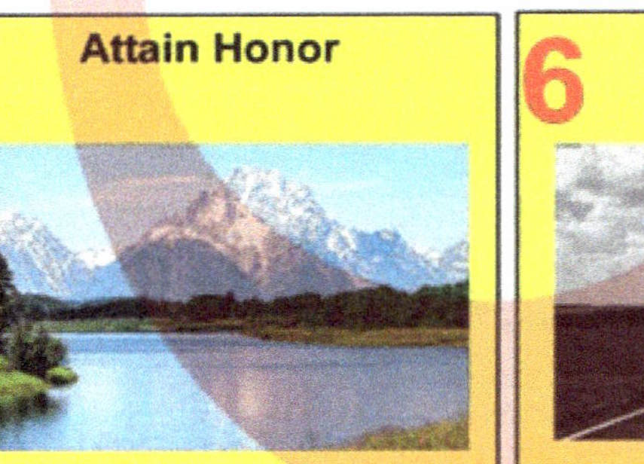

Live by principle - stand firm in what you believe, while allowing challenges to flow around you. Stand like a mountain, flow like a river.

6 Change Your Reality

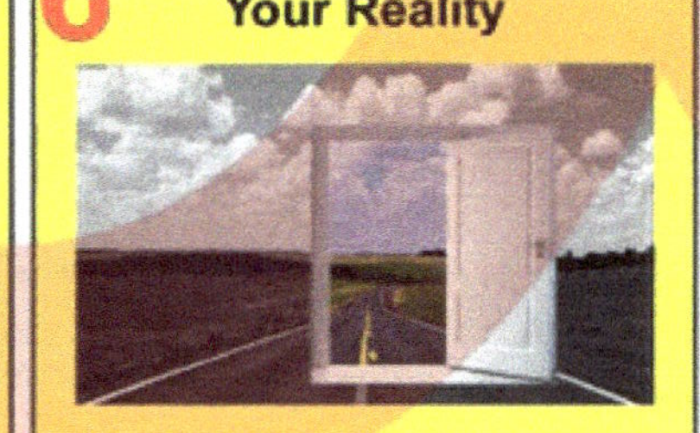

Understand that you are in control of your life and the choices you make determine your success or failure within your reality.

7 Become a Living Vessel of Wisdom

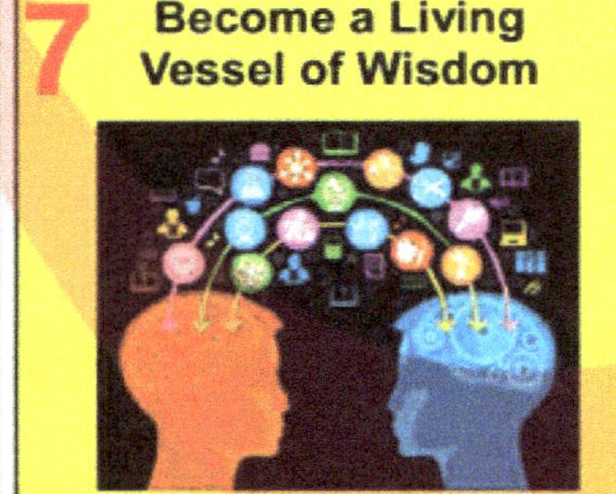

Knowledge alone is not power. The sharing of our knowledge, is when knowledge becomes powerful.

8 Draw on Nature's Power

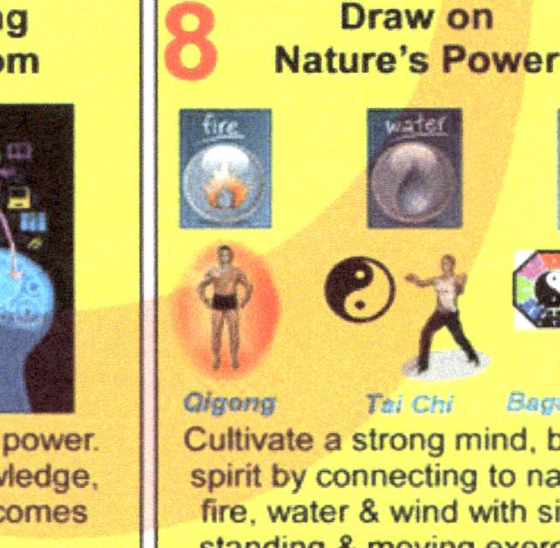

Cultivate a strong mind, body & spirit by connecting to nature's fire, water & wind with sitting, standing & moving exercises.

We are not our thoughts, but rather the observer and master of them. Within the Tao Te Ching we find the wisdom text relating to reflection in (Novak, 1994):

"Knowing others is intelligence,
knowing yourself is true wisdom.
Mastering others is strength,
mastering yourself is true power.
If you realize that you have enough,
you are truly rich..."

We can seek to find the root causes of turbidity and chaos in our society today, where most people do not aspire to see their true selves and the chaos coming from within. This can be evident in our lack of taking ownership and accountability for any of our own behaviors. Self-reflection is a very important component of any belief system or spiritual cultivation. It is called reflection because in ancient times, mirrors did not exist. One would actually have to look at water in order to see their own image or a reflection thereof. If the water was moving or turbid it would not be possible to see one's reflection. Similarly, if one's thoughts and relative lifestyle are turbid, it is very difficult for one to self-reflect. Your mind is that water and so you never really get a chance to see your true nature because it's not very tranquil enough and never clear enough to reveal even just a fleeting glimpse of our true nature. This is an important component of spirituality, self-improvement, self-awareness, or whatever one chooses to call this concept. This nature of *our* higher nature isn't just *your* nature. It is *my* nature. It is *his and her* nature. It is *all of our* nature. It is all the same nature being that we are all basically connected. The divine in me sees the divine in all. We all have one little particle of that highest nature and when it is momentarily separated, we suffer the illusion of individuality for only a moment.

I do not see Taoism, Confucianism, or Buddhism as religions, but rather as life philosophies in that they hold principles that can easily be seen and/or incorporated into other spiritual belief systems. What I find most appealing about Taoism is that I don't find it to be a religion by definition, but rather a philosophy of how to navigate the human condition. I have found that Taoism at its core seeks to focus on holistic, universal, and peaceful principles of living in harmony with nature and the natural order of all within it, whether alive or inanimate.

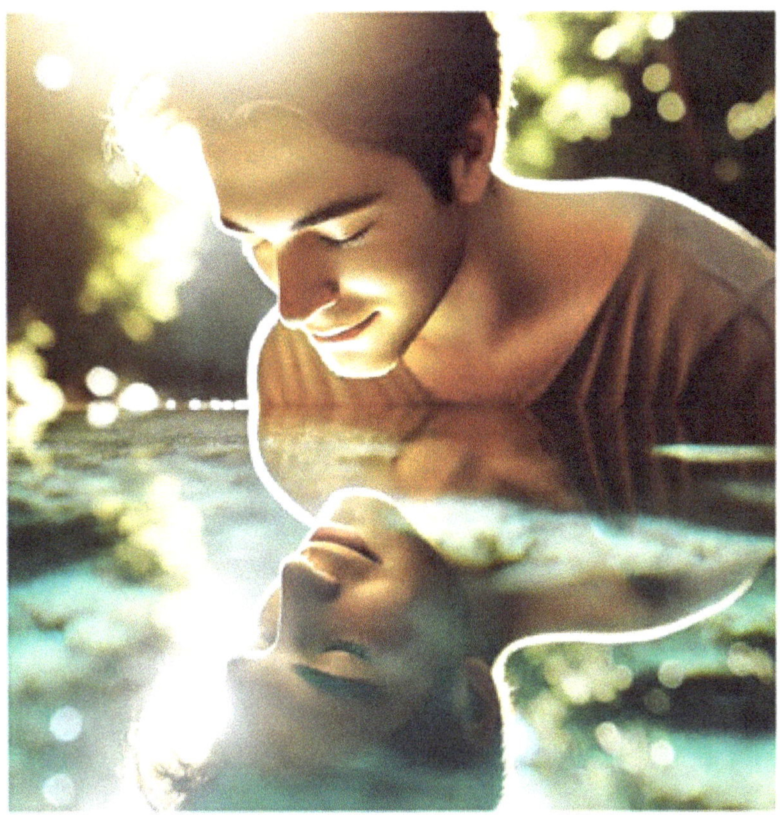

Strive to see your true nature

References

Chinese Religions and Philosophies | National Geographic Society. (2022, May 20). National Geographic. Retrieved August 9, 2022, from https://education.nationalgeographic.org/resource/chinese-religions-and-philosophies/

Hon, Tze-Ki, "Chinese Philosophy of Change (Yijing)", The Stanford Encyclopedia of Philosophy (Summer 2019 Edition), Edward N. Zalta (ed.), URL = https://plato.stanford.edu/archives/sum2019/entries/chinese-change

Novak, P. (1994). The World's Wisdom. Retrieved from https://platform.virdocs.com/r/s/0/doc/122387/sp/178876424/mi/570541808?cfi=%2F4%5Btext%5D%2F2%5Bchapter06%5D%2F6%2F250%2F2%2C%2F1%3A0%2C%2F1%3A0

Smith, H. (2009). The World's Religions. Retrieved from https://platform.virdocs.com/r/s/0/doc/119147/sp/178692013/mi/570158024?cfi=%2F4%2F2%5Bch8%5D%2F4%2F182%2C%2F1%3A0%2C%2F1%3A0

Wuxing (Wu-hsing) | Internet Encyclopedia of Philosophy. (n.d.). Internet Encyclopedia of Philosophy. Retrieved August 9, 2022, from https://iep.utm.edu/wuxing/

Part VI – Appendices

Glossary

Acupoints (Acupuncture Points)
Specific locations along meridians where Qi can be accessed, influenced, or regulated through touch, needles, or pressure.

Bagua (Eight Trigrams)
A Taoist symbolic system representing dynamic patterns of change, often used to describe energetic transformation and movement cycles.

Chong Mai (Penetrating Vessel)
An Extraordinary Vessel associated with deep constitutional energy, blood regulation, and emotional integration.

Dan Tian (Dantian)
Primary energy centers of the body (lower, middle, upper) where Qi is cultivated, stored, and refined.

Du Mai (Governing Vessel)
A central Extraordinary Vessel running along the spine, influencing the brain, nervous system, and Yang energy.

Emptiness (Xu)
A Taoist concept describing receptive openness or stillness; the internal "space" in which transformation of Jing, Qi, and Shen occurs.

Five Elements (Wu Xing)
A system describing Wood, Fire, Earth, Metal, and Water as dynamic phases governing physiological, emotional, and energetic processes.

Interoception
The ability to sense internal bodily states such as breath, heartbeat, and tension; foundational to somatic awareness.

Jing (Essence)
The foundational physical substance of life, associated with genetics, growth, and long-term vitality.

Jing Luo (Meridian Network)
The interconnected system of channels through which Qi and Blood circulate throughout the body.

Jing-Well Points
Acupoints located at the fingertips and toes, used to stimulate energy flow and restore consciousness or vitality.

Meridians (Primary Channels)
The 12 main pathways that circulate Qi and Blood, supporting organ function and systemic balance.

Nei Dan (Internal Alchemy)
Advanced Taoist practice focused on refining Jing → Qi → Shen through awareness, breath, and internal transformation.

Parasympathetic Nervous System
The "rest-and-digest" branch of the autonomic nervous system, activated through breath and relaxation practices.

Prenatal Qi (Yuan Qi)
Inherited life energy received from one's parents, stored primarily in the kidneys and foundational to vitality.

Proprioception
Awareness of body position and movement in space; essential for coordination and physical alignment.

Qi (Chi)
Vital life energy that animates all living systems; circulates through meridians and supports physiological and mental function.

Qi Flow
The movement and circulation of energy throughout the body; smooth flow indicates health, stagnation indicates imbalance.

Qigong (Chi Kung)
A system of breath, movement, and awareness practices designed to cultivate, regulate, and enhance Qi.

Ren Mai (Conception Vessel)
An Extraordinary Vessel running along the front midline of the body, associated with Yin energy and nourishment.

Shen (Spirit)
The refined aspect of consciousness, awareness, and presence; associated with clarity, insight, and higher integration.

Somatic Calibration
The process of tuning the body through awareness, posture, and breath to establish physiological stability and sensitivity.

Three Treasures (San Bao)
The foundational triad of Jing (essence), Qi (energy), and Shen (spirit), representing stages of human development and refinement.

Wei Qi (Defensive Qi)
Protective energy circulating at the surface of the body, defending against external pathogens and regulating temperature.

Wu Wei
A Taoist principle meaning “effortless action” or acting in harmony with natural flow rather than force.

Xu (Emptiness)
See *Emptiness*; the underlying field of potential and transformation in Taoist philosophy.

Yin and Yang
Complementary opposites that describe dynamic balance within all systems (e.g., rest/activity, cold/heat, internal/external).

Zang-Fu Organs
The organ systems in TCM, divided into Yin (Zang) and Yang (Fu), each with physiological and energetic functions.

About the Instructor, Author & Artist - Jim Moltzan

While this book includes supplemental resources, its primary aim is not instruction, but integration supporting readers in understanding how healing unfolds across body, mind, meaning, and lived life.

My fitness training started at the age of 16 and has continued for almost 45 years. During that time, I attended high school, then college, and worked 2 jobs all while pursuing further training in martial arts and other fitness methods. Many years ago, I started up an additional business to help finance my next goal of owning my own school. I moved to Florida from the Midwest to make this goal a reality. Having owned two wellness and martial arts schools, I have surpassed what I once believed to be my potential. At this stage in my life, I have chosen not to open any more schools, as I found the business aspects took too much focus away from my true passion: training and teaching others.

Beyond my professional endeavors, I am also a husband and father of two grown children. I believe that we must be prepared to work hard mentally, physically and financially to earn our good health and well-being. Not only for ourselves but for our families as well. Good health always comes at a cost whether in time, effort, cost, sacrifice or some combination of the previous.

I returned to college in my later 50's, to pursue my BS in Holistic Health (wellness and alternative medicine). My degree program covered many wide-ranging topics such as anatomy and physiology, meditation, massage, nutrition, herbology, chemistry, biology, history and basis of various medical modalities such as allopathic, Traditional Chinese Medicine, Ayurveda/yoga, naturopathy, chiropractic, and complimentary alternative methods. I also studied religion, mythology of the world, stress relief/management as well as sociology, psychology (human behavior) and cultural issues associated with better health and wellness.

Most of the movements I teach and write about originate from Chinese martial arts. The Qigong (breathing work) is from Chinese Kung Fu and the Korean Dong Han medical Qigong lineage. I have also gained much knowledge of Traditional Chinese Medicine (TCM) from many TCM practitioners, martial arts masters, teachers and peers. This includes many techniques and practices of acupressure (reflexology, auricular, Jing Well, etc.), acupuncture, moxibustion as well as preparation of some herbal remedies and extracts for conditioning and injuries. I have been studying for over 20 years with Zen Wellness, learning medical Qigong as well as other Eastern methods of fitness, philosophy and self-cultivation. I have been recognized as a "Gold Coin" master instructor having trained and taught others for at least 10000 hours or roughly over 35 years. The core fitness movements are from Kung Fu and its forms in Tai Chi, Baguazhang, Dao Yin and Ship Pal Gi (Korean Kung Fu and weapons training). Each martial art has mental, physical and spiritual aspects that can complement and enhance one another. The more ways that you can move your body and engage your mind, the better it is for your overall health.

Physical health, mental well-being and the relationships within our lives; are these the most cherished aspects of our existence? Yet, how much effort do we put towards improving these areas on a daily basis? Many have used martial arts and other mind-body methods of training as methods of learning to see one's character as others see them. I feel that I can offer the priceless qualities of truth, honor and integrity with my instruction. You must seek the right teacher for you, because in time a student can become similar to their teacher. Through the training that I have experienced and offer to others, an individual can understand and hopefully reach their full potential.

By developing self-discipline to continuously execute and perfect sets of movements, an individual can start to understand not only how they work physically but also mentally and emotionally. You can find your strengths and your weaknesses and improve them both. Through disciplined training, one not only enhances physical abilities but also cultivates mental resilience, allowing them to achieve their fullest potential in all areas of life.

I have co-authored a book, produced numerous other books and journals, graphic charts and study guides related to the mind and body connection and how it relates to martial arts, fitness, and self-improvement. A few hundred of my classes and lectures are viewable on YouTube.com.

Lineage

- Recognized as a 1000 and 10,000-hour student and teacher
- Earned gold coins through the Doh Yi Masters and Zen Wellness program
- Earned a 5th degree in Korean Kung Fu through the Dong Han lineage

Education

Bachelor of Science in Holistic Medicine - Vermont State University

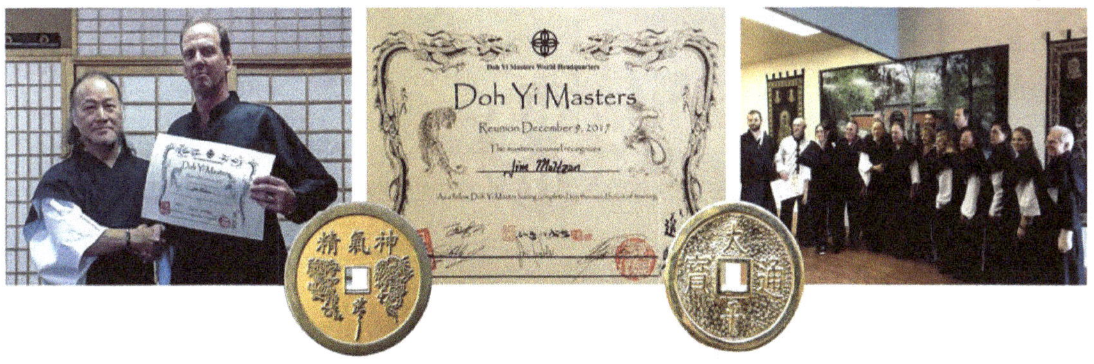

Books Available Through Amazon

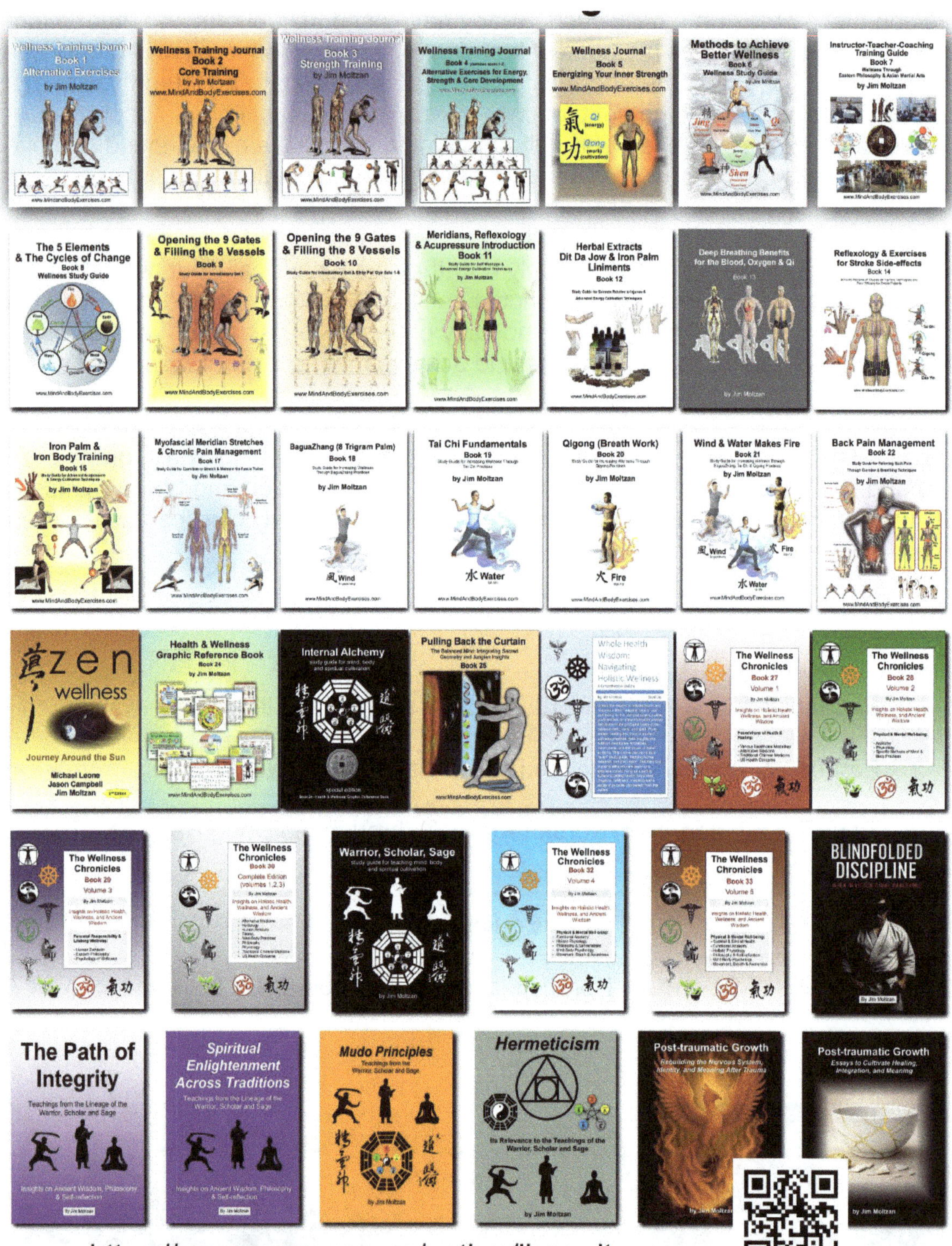

https://www.amazon.com/author/jimmoltzan

Book Titles by Jim Moltzan

Book 1 - Alternative Exercises
Book 2 - Core Training
Book 3 - Strength Training
Book 4 - Combo of 1-3
Book 5 - Energizing Your Inner Strength
Book 6 - Methods to Achieve Better Wellness
Book 7 - Coaching & Instructor Training Guide
Book 8 - The 5 Elements & the Cycles of Change
Book 9 - Opening the 9 Gates & Filling 8 Vessels-Intro Set 1
Book 10 - Opening the 9 Gates & Filling 8 Vessels-sets 1 to 8
Book 11 - Meridians, Reflexology & Acupressure
Book 12 - Herbal Extracts, Dit Da Jow & Iron Palm Liniments
Book 13 - Deep Breathing Benefits for the Blood, Oxygen & Qi
Book 14 - Reflexology for Stroke Side Effects:
Book 15 - Iron Body & Iron Palm
Book 17 - Fascial Train Stretches & Chronic Pain Management
Book 18 - BaguaZhang
Book 19 - Tai Chi Fundamentals
Book 20 - Qigong (breath-work)
Book 21 - Wind & Water Make Fire
Book 22 - Back Pain Management
Book 23 - Journey Around the Sun-2nd Edition
Book 24 - Graphic Reference Book
Book 25 - Pulling Back the Curtain
Book 26 - Whole Health Wisdom: Navigating Holistic Wellness
Book 27 - The Wellness Chronicles (volume 1)
Book 28 - The Wellness Chronicles (volume 2)
Book 29 - The Wellness Chronicles (volume 3)
Book 30 - The Wellness Chronicles (complete edition, volumes 1-3)
Book 31 - Warrior, Scholar, Sage
Book 32 - The Wellness Chronicles (volume 4)
Book 33 - The Wellness Chronicles (volume 5)
Book 34 - Blindfolded Discipline
Book 35 - The Path of Integrity

Book 36 - Spiritual Enlightenment Across Traditions
Book 37 - Mudo Principles: Teachings from the Warrior, Scholar, and Sage
Book 38 – Hermeticism -Its Relevance to the Teachings of the Warrior, Scholar and Sage
Book 39 - Post Traumatic Growth
Book 40 - Post Traumatic Growth - Essays to Cultivate Healing, Integration, and Meaning
Book 41 - Architecture of the Human Journey – The Self-Healing Body
Book 42 - Architecture of the Human Journey – The Biological Mind
Book 43 - Architecture of the Human Journey – The Energetic Body
Book 44 - Architecture of the Human Journey – Embodied Discipline
Book 45 - Architecture of the Human Journey – The Healthcare Paradox
Book 46 - Architecture of the Human Journey – The Human Journey

https://www.amazon.com/author/jimmoltzan

For more information regarding charts, products, classes and instruction:

Website

www.MindAndBodyExercises.com
info@MindAndBodyExercises.com

www.youtube.com/c/MindandBodyExercises
www.MindAndBodyExercises.wordpress.com

Blog

407-234-0119

Social Media:

Facebook: MindAndBodyExercises
Instagram: MindAndBodyExercises
Twitter: MindAndBodyExercise

YouTube Channel

Jim Moltzan - Mind and Body Exercises
522 Hunt Club Blvd. #305
Apopka, FL 32703

www.ingramcontent.com/pod-product-compliance
Lightning Source LLC
LaVergne TN
LVHW081409110826
845149LV00010B/1683

* 9 7 8 1 9 5 8 8 3 7 5 7 3 *